CONSTIPAT
KICK IT NATURALLY

By
T.C. Hale
& Two Other Guys

Copyright © 2017 Words to Spare, LLC. All rights reserved, including the right to reproduce this book, or portions thereof, in any form. No part of the text may be reproduced, transmitted, downloaded, decompiled, reverse engineered, or stored in or introduced into any information storage and retrieval system, in any form or by any means, whether electronic or mechanical without the express written permission of the author. (Unless you're getting a tattoo and want to tattoo part of my book on your body. That is okay.) The scanning, uploading, and distribution of this book via the Internet or via any other means without the permission of the publisher is illegal and punishable by law. I will also speak poorly of you on my blog. Please purchase only authorized electronic editions, and do not participate in or encourage electronic piracy or copyrighted material.

Cover Designed by T.C. Hale & Arthur Angelo

Copyright © Words to Spare, LLC 2017

File Version 1.01.1

For Mom, if only someone had taught me this earlier.

WHAT THE CELEBRITIES SAY

"Working with Tony is like jumping into the arms of your favorite aunt. Except it's not. At all. I mean, his methods work. But it's not like that at all." - **Jane Lynch (*Glee*)**

"I confess to being a full-blown 'gymophobe.' (I still have flashbacks of my mean fourth-grade gym teacher!) Tony actually makes the gym panic-attack free." - **Tom Kenny (Voice of Spongebob)**

"Wait. You mean the short skinny trainer dude with the neon sneakers who writes books about women's menstrual cramps? Did he ever get a single menstrual cramp? I don't think so. The guy who helps fat people get skinnier? Was he ever fat? I don't think so. And what's with the whole fake I don't talk thing? Is it turrets? If he did talk, would it be a string of expletives even I would be offended by? I guess he has a sense of humor. That's something good." - **Betty Thomas (Director: 28 *Days*, *The Brady Bunch Movie*, etc.)**

"You can argue with Tony, or you can do what he says and buy smaller jeans." - **Kari Wahlgren (Voice of Tigress, *Kung Fu Panda: Legends of Awesomeness*)**

"Tony took on my Jewish-Cuban hips and he won! He let me pretend the punching bag was my ex's mom. That was fun and I got in shape too. I adore him but my tush loves him more." - **Brigitte Bako (*G Spot*, *The Red Shoe Diaries*)**

"I always look forward to my weekly beatings from Tony." - **Tucker Barkley (Dance Choreographer: *The X Factor*)**

"So you know that moment when you are just finishing a hard workout with Tony and he says, 'Alright, you warmed up? We can start now?' and then he laughs... I hate that moment." - **Kayla Radomski (*So You Think You Can Dance*)**

ACKNOWLEDGEMENTS

Thank you to my co-authors and collaborators. Without your help and patience, this book would still be a big stack of ideas.

Thank you to my readers, editors and contributors: Alex and Red Donnally, Nina Florez, Elaine Alcala, and James Singleton.

Thank you to my brother, Richard, who is also an author, for his insight into how to not be a sucky author. I don't understand why you haven't checked out his books yet. He writes great thrillers.

www.RichardCHaleAuthor.com

Finally, I'd like to thank you, the reader, for allowing me to entertain myself throughout this book, instead of just getting to the point, even though you may want to poop right now. I thank you for indulging me.

Big Flippin' Disclaimer

This book is not intended as a substitute for the medical recommendations of a physician or other healthcare provider. Don't be stupid. It's just a book. This book is intended to entertain and to offer information to help the reader cooperate with physicians and health professionals in a mutual quest of improved well-being.

The identities of people described in this book have been changed to protect confidentiality. Even when I talk about John Tesh. That could be a totally different John Tesh than the one you might be thinking of.

The Kick It Naturally series is written and published as an information resource and educational guide for both professionals and non-professionals. It should not be used to replace medical advice.

The publisher and the author are not responsible for any goods and/or services offered or referred to in this book and expressly disclaim all liability in connection with the fulfillment of orders for any such goods and/or services and for any damages, loss, or expense to person or property arising out of or relating to them. You are responsible for your own health and wellness.

Please Visit the Author's Website at:

www.KickItNaturally.com

Website for Health Professionals
www.SixFigureHealthPro.com

Or follow him on Twitter and Facebook:

www.twitter.com/KickItInTheNuts
www.facebook.com/KickItInTheNuts
www.facebook.com/KickItNaturally

TABLE OF CONTENTS

CONSTIPATION
KICK IT NATURALLY   I

What The Celebrities Say   iv

Acknowledgements   v

Big Flippin' Disclaimer   vi

Please Visit the Author's Website at: vii

Important Introduction   14
    How To Use This Book   14
    About The Author   15

Chapter One   20
    Hi   20
    Slackers and Geniuses Unite   22
    Why Am I Reading A Natural Health Book Written By A Comedian?   23
    About This Series Of Books   23
    Take The Quiz   25
    A New Light On Health   26
    How Medications Work   27
    Getting The Most From This Book   28
    Testing Tools You'll Need For This Book   29
    Wha'd He Say?   31

Chapter Two   32
    Seriously? I Just Wanna Poop!   32
    What's Behind Constipation?   32
    Why Can't I Poop? All My Friends Poop.   33
    It's Not About Fiber And Probiotics   33
    What Causes The Cork?   34

Water's Role In Constipation	35
My Mother And Grandmother Were Constipated Too	35
I Can Fix This?	36
Understanding Digestion Can Help You Tweak Your Digestion	37
Working With A Health Coach	38
What To Expect	38
Wha'd He Say?	38

Chapter Three — 40

Digestion	40
Everything Goes Back To Digestion	40
How's Your Digestion?	41
The Digestive Summary	42
Give Me Acid Or Give Me Death	44
Improving Your Stomach Acid	45
You Need Good Bile Flow	49
Improving Your Bile Flow	49
Add Digestive Enzymes	50
Where To Get Supplements	51
Supplements Review	52
Wha'd He Say?	52

Chapter Four — 54

Elimination & Digestion Gone Wild	54
Let's Talk Poop	54
Burping, Bloating And Passing Gas	55
Helping Your Liver	56
Is Constipation Making Me Gain Weight?	57
Conquering Our Food - Food Allergies and Sensitivities	58
Acid Reflux, GERD, & Heartburn	60
Wha'd He Say?	60

Chapter Five — 61

Simple Self-Testing	61
This Is The Magic	61
Data Tracking Sheet	63
The Coalition	65
Let's Get To Testing...	66
Simple Testing Procedures	67

pH of Urine and Saliva	68
Blood Pressure	70
Breath Rate	70
Breath Hold Time	71
Bonus Test - Blood Glucose	71
Easy Peasy	72
Wha'd He Say?	72

Chapter Six — 73
Understanding Your Biological Individuality	73
Intro To Imbalances	73
Imbalance Guide	76
Conclusions	83
Wha'd He Say?	84

Chapter Seven — 85
How Imbalances Contribute To Constipation	85
Electrolyte State	85
Catabolic/Anabolic States	90
Energy Production	93
Using The Coalition	94
Improving Imbalances	96
Wha'd He Say?	97

Chapter Eight — 98
What Else Can Help?	98
Fiber	98
Water	99
Avoid Soda	100
Lose The Artificial Sweeteners	101
Use Unrefined Salt (Sea Salt)	103
Knowledge	103
Simma Down Now	105
Wha'd He Say?	106

Chapter Nine — 107
Foods Specific To You	107
Eat Real Food	107
Diet Is Determined By Strength Of Digestion	108

Foods That Could Help	108
Contradictions From Imbalance To Imbalance	111
Imbalance - Electrolyte Excess	114
Imbalance – Anabolic	115
Imbalance – Catabolic	116
Imbalance - Carb Burner	117
Imbalance - Fat Burner	118
Wha'd He Say?	119

Chapter Ten — 120

Supplements That Could Help	120
Finding Effective Supplements	120
What If I Hate Taking Supplements?	122
Digestive Supplement Review	123
Fiber	124
Constipation All Stars	124
Improving Imbalances Through Supplementation	124
Imbalance - Electrolyte Deficiency	126
Imbalance - Electrolyte Excess	127
Imbalance – Anabolic	128
Imbalance – Catabolic	129
Imbalance - Carb Burner	130
Imbalance - Fat Burner	130
Major Constipation Supplement Winners and Who Should Use Them	130
Finding A Qualified Health Coach In Your Area	137
Wha'd He Say?	137

Chapter Eleven — 138

Case Studies & FAQs	138
Case Study: Jan	145
FAQs	148
Referencing These FAQs	152
Wha'd He Say?	153

Chapter Twelve (The Sum Up) — 154

Review & Make Your Plan	154
Now What?	154
Bring It All Together	154
Fix Digestive Issues	155

Correct Your Imbalances	156
Monitor Your Numbers	156
Don't Work Against Yourself	157
Make Your Plan	157
Avoid Screwing Yourself Over	158
Finding Supplements	161
Optimal Measurement Ranges	161
Continue To Learn	162
What Else Are You Struggling With?	162
Follow Me	162
Our Radio Show	163
Give Yourself A Reminder	163
Help Us Spread the Word or Become a Coach	163
Join The Community And Get Support	164
Be Excited	164
Final Words	164

Appendix A — 165

More Digestive Explanations	165
Reflux, Heartburn And GERD	165
Crohn's, Colitis, And IBS	167
Birth Control Medications	168
Gallbladder Removal / Gallstones / Olive Oil-Lemon Drink	169
H. Pylori Infections & Natural Protocols	172

Appendix B — 179

Intermediate Testing Procedures	179
Resting to Standing - Blood Pressure Test	180
Dermographic Line	181
Gag Reflex	181
Pupil Size	181
11-Parameter Urine Dipstick	182
Bonus Test - Hemochromatosis	184
Learn More	186
Sorting Out The Data	186
Imbalance Guide Content	187
Okay, I Can Add Check Marks... Now What?	191
Conclusions	193

Appendix C 194
    Imbalances 194
    Electrolyte State 194
    Catabolic/Anabolic States 197
    Energy Production 200
    Autonomic Nervous System 203
    pH Balance - Acid/Alkaline Imbalances 204
    Alkalizing Water And Water Filters 208

Appendix D 211
    Those Who Paved the Way 211
    Dr. Carey Reams 211
    Dr. Emanuel Revici 211
    Thomas Riddick 212
    Dr. Melvin Page 213
    Recommended Reading 213

Appendix E 214
    A Healthy Body In An Unhealthy World 214
    Chemicals In Tap Water 215
    Shower Filters 217
    Microwaves 218
    What Am I Cooking In? 219
    What's In My Mouth? 219
    Smoking 220
    Antibiotics 220
    Flu Shots 221
    Alkalizing Water And Water Filters 221

More About Tony 222

References 224

IMPORTANT INTRODUCTION

How To Use This Book

If this is your first time reading one of my books, you may be very pleasantly surprised by what you find in these pages. I hear from readers every day who are shocked that it took a comedian to supply them with answers they have been searching for years to find. After bouncing from one healthcare professional to another for months, or even a lifetime, most people don't expect a book from a comic to uncover health solutions that are easy to understand. These readers are often even more shocked when those solutions actually work.

You may even be one of those readers I'm talking about and you're now reading this book to learn more about constipation. If you have read any of my other books, some content of this book (as well as some of the jokes) may sound familiar to you. For example, digestion is so important when dealing with such a variety of issues, the chapter on digestion winds up in nearly all of my books. Much of this book will teach you how to look at you and your chemistry. Knowing your own chemistry is the most important factor when dealing with any health issue. In each of my books, I have given readers a foundation of information about chemical imbalances in the body, how to test their own chemistry, and how to view the information they find through testing. Those tools and methods reveal what is important no matter what health issue you would like to see improve. If you already have a good understanding of those techniques from one of my other books, you'll be miles ahead and you will be able to use this title to better understand how specific imbalances can relate to constipation.

To better understand many health problems, you may not even need to read our other books or wait for us to write a book on the issue you'd like to improve. We have covered a wide variety of health topics on our *Kick It Naturally* podcast. Once this book teaches you how to get a better idea of imbalances you may be dealing with, the podcast could help you better understand why specific health issues may have shown up and the steps that might bring about a good result for you. For example, if you deal with seasonal allergies, you may be able to listen to our episode on that topic to get a better idea of how different imbalances can exacerbate allergies. Coupling what you learn in this book with additional information on the podcast episodes may turn out to be a wealth of information for you and your family.

If you've already taken one of my advanced health coach courses, or you've read enough of my other work to have a full understanding of digestion, imbalances, and how the body works, you might be able to skip a lot of the content where I explain all the foundational basics to those reading these ideas for the first time. For my advanced students, I will put all foundational content (the content you would have already read if you've read any of my other books), in a gray box. You might be able to skip those sections if you're a veteran T.C. Hale reader.

If you're a first time reader, when you see a section in a gray box, know that the material in that section is some of the most important in the entire book. As you'll soon learn, to improve any health symptom, you must first understand what is causing that symptom for you. Since just about every problem (like constipation), can have more than one underlying cause, to figure out how to improve your constipation, you first must understand how your unique body is operating.

For these foundational sections that appear in almost all of our books, I use this "gray box" formatting to help these sections stand out more. If you decide to read more of my books, this system will help you distinguish issue-specific information from the foundational topics you will have already read in this book. I will use my personal introduction as an example of this "foundational content" formatting.

About The Author

Before we get to the science, let me first explain why you're reading a natural health book from a comedian. My name is Tony Hale. I use the pen name "T.C. Hale" because if you Google "Tony Hale" you find four hundred thousand pictures of Buster Bluth from *Arrested Development*. If you're unfamiliar with the actor, one of his first big national spots was that Volkswagen commercial with the guy doing the robot in his car. I can remember studying at The Groundlings (an Improv school that churns out a lot of *SNL* players) when a girl in my class told me that her friend's name was Tony Hale too, and that he was the guy in the Volkswagen commercial. I recall thinking, "That bastard's going to call dibs on my name before I do," and that's pretty much how it worked out. I run into Tony around town from time to time and he's actually a super nice guy. The first time I met him, he was shopping at Whole Foods. I walked up to him, didn't say a word, and just handed him my driver's license. "No way!" he said after seeing my name.

Turns out, he was excited to meet me because he had heard of my existence since I have an acting credit that is listed on his IMDb.com page. When I was touring as a comic, I was dating a girl who booked one of the leads in an independent film called *Raging Hormones*. Visiting her on set, the director asked me to drive by in a scene and make fun of the main character. It earned me a film credit, but they attached it to the wrong Tony Hale. Since this was literally THE worst movie that has ever been created, I decided to let Tony keep the credit. But, enough about my name already. What about the rest? How the hell did I get here?

I guess like most natural health and nutrition researchers, my background comes from a professional career in stand-up comedy. I became a natural health and nutrition researcher by necessity. On Valentine's Day 2003, I took my girlfriend at the time to see The Dan Band at the club, Hollywood and Highland. Most of the night, I talked over the loud music. The next day, my voice was gone and it didn't come back. Over the next year or so, 23 doctors, specialists, and surgeons couldn't figure out what the problem was. With each doctor and each medication, my health seemed to decline a little more. After exhausting my way through doctors, speech therapists, natural practitioners, and a six-figure accumulation of expenses, I told everybody to piss off and decided I was going to figure this out myself.

And that's what I did. Over the next six years I did nothing but read books, research nutrition experts, and attend workshops and seminars across the country. As I searched for my own answers, I kept stumbling across answers to problems that my friends were dealing with. I was so amazed to find explanations that I had never heard of that I started to share them with my friends. When I emailed my buddy Greg and explained to him some of the underlying issues that can make a person have to sit on the toilet twelve times a day, he ran some measurements on himself to see what the likely causes were and his chemistry matched up perfectly with most people who have similar issues. He tried the things I showed him and he was able to poop like a normal human, once or twice a day, instead of shooting soup out the back door all day.

As one friend would tell another friend, people kept emailing me and asking if I could help them understand their health issues. But I was working as a personal trainer and didn't have time to teach all those people how to look at their own chemistry to understand why they're dealing with what they're dealing with. That is, until a guy named Jim, who was so impressed with how I taught his friend how to understand and improve his insomnia, offered me $500 to help him, too. That's when I realized, "Oh, this is a business." After all, I would have gladly paid someone $10,000 to help me correct my issue years earlier. That's a lot of money, but it still would have saved me $90,000 and reduced the six years it took for me to start getting my voice back. With this revelation, I started a career as a health coach. I've never advertised, but today I help some of the biggest stars and most influential people in the entertainment industry better understand how they can use nutrition to improve their health. That is also what I'm going to do with you in these pages. Isn't that nice of me? You don't even have your own show and I'm still going to help you.

Before you look at anything I have to say as gospel, I want to make sure that I am very clear on the fact that I am not a doctor and I don't claim to be any sort of doctor or licensed professional. I don't even watch *House*. I used to think M*A*S*H was funny, but that hardly makes me a doctor. What I am is a guy who became fed up with the system and decided I would find my answers elsewhere. I'm just a guy who had no choice but to keep digging until solutions were uncovered. I had no choice because it was becoming clear that I wasn't going to be able to talk again unless I found real answers. If it were anything else, I probably would have given up after two years. For example, if I were just walking with a limp, or I couldn't talk without whistling and spitting on people, or whatever the case may be, I probably would have just learned to live with it. But since I was very determined to get my voice back, I was willing to do the work. Remember, a stand-up comic with no voice is just a mime—and who wants to get punched in the face while they're working every day? You may not know this, but it has been statistically proven that 83% of the population would rather punch a mime than watch him try to entertain a crowd. Since I was so determined not to become another "mime statistic," you now get to reap the rewards of my years of research.

So, if you're looking for credentials, buy another book. I encountered plenty of professionals with credentials, certifications, licenses, awards, accolades, expensive offices... you name it. One guy even had a live ostrich that lived in the backyard of his office complex. (That didn't help, either.) The professionals I consulted had it all. Yet, none of them could help me. As a result of that experience, I find that I'm more interested in the truth than I am in credentials. Over the last 60 years, doctor after doctor who went outside the box to try to truly help patients (by working to correct the actual causes of their illnesses instead of just treating symptoms) have been stripped of their licenses, discredited, and basically run out of town. Sadly, this happens frequently. It seems like every time someone makes a significant splash in the mainstream market with any advances that could help people correct health issues naturally, that individual is discredited so that the masses will go back to spending billions on drugs that only mask their symptoms.

With these *Kick It Naturally* books, since my co-authors and I know this information will spread fast, we're going to go another route. After all, when people finally get answers to problems they have been dealing with for decades, they talk about it. So we're setting up a system where people can learn about their body without having that system discredited. It can't be discredited because I am the voice and I'm telling you right now, I HAVE NO CREDENTIALS. I'm just a schmuck comedian and personal trainer who was willing to dig for his own answers. And now I'm sharing what I've learned with you, so you can dig for your answers a little quicker. Am I a doctor? No. Do I have a license? Heck no. Do we really need one more person following the same system that isn't working? I don't even shave every day, I've filed for bankruptcy in my life, I don't understand what color shirt I'm allowed to wear with brown pants, and I'm writing this book in my boxers.

Though I am not the only author in this series of books, I have been elected to be the voice and will be the only known author for many of our titles. In this book, as well as others in this series, my co-authors and contributors are made up of doctors, M.D.s, medical and natural health researchers, and some of the most well respected educators who teach doctors from all over the world about nutrition. When I traveled the country looking for answers, I found a number of individuals who have dedicated their lives to this work. I've approached many of them to help me in this effort. Though some have chosen to have their names added as co-authors to a number of our titles, many are keeping their identity anonymous, so as to protect their practices and keep the powers-that-be from trying to discredit the amazing work they are doing. One name I can share with you is Will Wolfgang Schmidt. If you've listened to our *Kick It Naturally* show, you're familiar with Will. Will is a celebrity trainer, one of the co-hosts on our show, and helps me do a lot of research for books like this one. You'll see a lot of Will if you end up watching any of our videos or taking any of our online courses.

Although I won't be sharing the names of most of my co-authors with you, I will share the pioneers from the 1930s and 1940s who first discovered these truths. That was the one constant that I seemed to find no matter who I talked to. Most of the experts I found had studied doctors from the 30s, 40s and 50s, back when a doctor was allowed to think. I'll talk about the work of these pioneers throughout our time together, and I'll even point you in the direction of some of their amazing books so you can dig deeper if you find this information as interesting as I did.

Odds are someone who experienced incredible results recommended this book to you. So, my suggestion is for you to put your trust in the experience of your friend instead of the authorities that seem to be more interested in profit than results. After all, wasn't it Benjamin Franklin who once said, "Though I have welcomed the words from authorities my whole life, it might be time for them to go flog themselves," or something like that?

CHAPTER ONE

Hi

It appears that you have come to me with a reasonable request. By buying this book, you are asking me, "Tony, may I please poop every day like a normal human being?" Seems like an odd request to ask someone you've never met. Nonetheless, I still feel like this is a reasonable request. I don't feel like you should have to watch with envy while your friends and family come out of the bathroom with smiles on their faces.

Maybe your only goal is to empty your bowels without the aid of six different laxatives, a sack full of fiber and an Indian rain dance. I understand. I've experienced constipation first hand and I'll be honest with you: I vote against it.

If I were to ask you to list the remedies you have tried in an effort to relieve your constipation, I bet you could fill the rest of this book. My guess is that you could also list remedies that worked for your friends but had little to no effect for you. Here's the big secret: there is no remedy for chronic constipation. Since constipation can have a variety of underlying causes, there will never be one solution that works for everyone.

Don't worry, that's not the end of this book. I would receive a whole bunch of violent emails if that were the case. However, in this book we're not going to waste time looking for "the remedy" for constipation. Instead, I'm going to have you focus on what will improve *your* constipation.

I know that you have ingested more fiber than should be legally allowed. I'm sure you're tired of eating beans to no avail. I know that you have tried probiotics until the cows came home. And when the cows got home, their first question was: Do you have anything to eat other than beans? Instead of packing you full of fiber, probiotics and herbal mixtures, the goal for you will be to understand why you're constipated in the first place. When you get a grip on what is clogging you up, it will just be a matter of doing the work to pop the cork. Wouldn't that be something?

If you've been dealing with chronic constipation for a long time, or even if this is a new hassle in your life, my co-authors and I will help you understand some of the actual causes behind constipation and teach you how other people have been correcting those causes for years. People all over the world are learning how they can look at their own physiology and understand their biological individuality. These people are learning about nutritional and lifestyle changes, specific to their body, that can help them poop like they mean business. And they're doing it without the help of laxatives or medications.

Since it is widely accepted that there are people who "simply don't go to the bathroom that often," and "that's just the way it is," I find that my clients are always surprised when they find answers to questions like:

How can I figure out which food choices are best for me?

Why is my stool so hard?

Why do I often have days without a bowel movement at all?

Why am I constipated one day and have diarrhea the next?

Why is the public so misguided about constipation?

My co-authors and I agree that, for the most part, the common answers to these questions are all over the map. The reality is this: It's not that nobody has the right answers, it's that nobody is asking the right questions. Not that I've fully examined every constipation remedy out there—I doubt that would even be humanly possible—but it is my experience that every remedy on the planet can work... for SOMEBODY. However, no remedy will work for EVERYBODY. It's not really about finding a remedy. It's more about moving your body into a state where it can function a little more optimally.

When it comes to constipation, the popular approach is to attack that symptom. The same holds true for any topic on health. A person is branded by symptoms. Do shoes come only in one size? How about bras or even contact lenses? No. We look at people as individuals for just about anything they need, except their health. In the world of healthcare, we're a one-trick pony. We're like a 7-11 that sells only Skittles. We look only at the symptoms instead of looking at the person who is suffering from the symptoms. And when our great, great grandkids learn about our health care system in their history classes, they will laugh at us. They will point, and they will laugh... and our only excuse will be that the characters on *Grey's Anatomy* were so dreamy, we just believed everything they said.

Constipation: Kick It Naturally was written to help you look at your own biological identity, understand how your specific body is operating, and make the necessary changes to help your body function in a more optimal way... so you can use your toilet for more than just a place to sit while you paint your toes.

Slackers and Geniuses Unite

Everyone is invited to join in. You're going to have the chance to decide what you want to get out of this book. You'll have the opportunity to begin implementing what you learn from the very beginning. Some of you will discover life-changing information and learn how to implement that knowledge within the first few chapters. You may be able to improve your constipation using what you've learned without ever reading past chapter six.

I'd also like to welcome any geniuses and those crazy people who read about something scientific and feel like they need to learn about every single aspect. That was me (the crazy person, not the genius). I became quite the researching maniac once I realized there were real answers out there. For you folks, I've included some pretty sciency stuff and I'll provide more in-depth explanations in the appendix section of the book. If you still want to learn more, you can also look into our advanced online Health Pro Course, at www.HealthProCourse.com. This course digs deeper into physiology and how nutrition can be used to improve your health.

Not everybody wants to understand the science. It wouldn't be the first time someone has said to me, "Hey Monkey Boy, just tell me what to do and I'll do it." With that in mind, know that you will have the choice of using the easy-to-follow methods in this book to improve your woes, or you can dig into all aspects of this book and gain a new understanding about nutrition, the human body, and why health issues are so common today.

Why Am I Reading A Natural Health Book Written By A Comedian?

While working at a seafood restaurant as a teenager, I once found a nickel inside a raw oyster. A nickel! It was as if the oyster was saving up to buy a pearl because nobody told him he was supposed to make his own. Well, in the same way that you can find something beautiful—like a pearl—in something so gross and snot-looking—like an oyster—you can also find something unexpected—like a nickel. My point is, I was surprised to find cash inside an oyster, but I was still able to use the cash on my way home that night when I stopped by the Taco Bell drive-through. So, just because you find information on natural health in a place you might not expect, that doesn't mean it can't be useful to you. My nickel helped pay for a Meximelt with no pico sauce, which was very useful to me.

I studied nutrition for twenty years before I came across the information I am sharing with you in this book. I truly thought I knew what I was talking about when it came to nutrition; but since I had my own health issues that were plaguing me, I was forced to do a tremendous amount of research on my own—and I was shocked at what I discovered. Now, you're about to benefit from my need to dig for real answers for myself. As it turns out, many of the keys to health are also the keys to proper bowel elimination, and vice versa.

About This Series Of Books

In the *Kick It Naturally* series of natural health books, I'll be helping you look at your health, body, and nutrition in a way that is different from any other natural health book you've ever read. Instead of just looking at a condition and talking about all the "natural remedies" that have been known to work for that condition, we're going to spend most of our time looking at YOU—the individual. Focusing only on the condition or symptoms is the biggest mistake in the world of health. It's like focusing on the straw that broke the camel's back instead of seeing the inordinate load that needs to be lifted off. With this series of books, it is my goal to offer you other options.

The truth is, every symptom or condition can have three or four different underlying causes. That's why so many "remedies" or methods will work great for one person with a particular symptom, but will make another person with the same symptom much worse. Rarely is anyone looking at each individual and the actual cause of the symptom for *that* individual.

I placed a disclaimer at the beginning of this book stating that this information should not replace any medical advice, etc, etc. Let's look a little deeper into this topic so you can have an understanding of what you might get out of this book. I don't want you to look at this book like it's going to be a tool to "beat your constipation." It's never a good idea to focus on trying to eliminate, declare war on, cure, or obliviate any problem. But once you see the direction the knowledge in this book can take you, you will see that trying to "beat" something is very rarely successful. Instead, the goal here is to teach you about the body's operational systems and what imbalances might be pushing in the wrong direction when common symptoms, like constipation, show up. Then I'm going to show you steps that others have taken in order to move their bodies back to a more balanced operational state. If you understand this objective, you will see that the goal should be to move toward health instead of trying to escape from, or beat down, symptoms or "disease."

Look at it this way... if you're in a dark, locked closet, there is nothing but darkness. You can't destroy the darkness. You can't beat it down or even run from it. To put your effort into changing that darkness into something else would be very frustrating and time consuming and your friends would say, "Hey, you've been in that closet for a long time... what the hell are you doing in there?" But if you turn on a light, the darkness will disappear on its own. Darkness cannot exist in a place where there is light. You didn't have to do anything to convince the darkness to leave or to stop tormenting you, you just invited something else into the closet that made it impossible for the darkness to exist there. You invited in the light and the darkness went away on its own.

Take The Quiz

If you have not already taken this quiz online or had a friend email it to you, take the time to answer these eight questions now. If you answer YES to any of the following questions, acquiring information about your body's biological individuality could be life-transforming. If you answer YES to many or most of the following questions, you might want to carry this book with you wherever you go—at least until you can answer NO to most of them. Many of the topics covered in this quiz are experienced by a large percentage of the population and these people walk through life believing this is just the way it is. By the time you finish this book, you will know that is not the case. You will know that the issues below can see improvement in almost any individual who is willing to put forth the effort. Good luck on your quiz, I know I didn't really let you prepare in any way. I always hated the teacher that would pull stunts like that.

(1) Do you ever go an entire day without a bowel movement?
    YES   NO
(2) Was your answer to the last question such an emphatic yes, that it required additional cussing?
    YES   NO
(3) Do you require the aid of laxatives or other natural remedies to experience consistent bowel movements?
    YES   NO
(4) Do you often burp after meals or feel bloated? (Even just small burps.)
    YES   NO
(5) Does your meal ever feel like it's sitting in your stomach like a rock for too long?
    YES   NO
(6) Is your stool normally hard and difficult to move?
    YES   NO
(7) Do you ever experience acid reflux or heartburn?
    YES   NO
(8) Do you commonly have to get up at night to pee?
    YES   NO

How did you do? If you can answer no to all of those questions, you may qualify to read this book for the jokes and then pass it along to a friend. But if you answered yes to one or more of those questions, you will likely have some life-long mysteries solved for yourself by the time you get to chapter six. That's a pretty fun reward considering you just failed the first pop quiz you've had since the tenth grade.

A New Light On Health

Let's get started by putting down a foundation. That foundation is to answer the questions that will run through your head for the duration of this book. "Why have I never heard this stuff? Why didn't my doctor tell me this when he pointed out that "some people don't poop very often, and that's just the way it is." Is nothing in this book true or does my doctor hate me?"

While digging for answers, there was one topic that really changed the way I looked at my health, the choices I was making, and where I wanted to find help. Before I explain this, I just want to be clear that in no way am I saying that the entire medical world is a crapshoot, or that the entire system is more evil than that blonde guy from *The Karate Kid*. The advances and information that medical professionals and researchers have provided are truly amazing and many of them do indeed save and/or prolong lives. Even some medications that result in horrible side effects still provide you with the ability to buy yourself some time and fight off a certain death long enough to really improve your health or correct the underlying problem. The only knock on how the whole system works that I cover here is this: We are given only half the story.

With that in mind, here's the piece of information I came across again and again while I was trying to figure out why each doctor and each medication was making me worse instead of better. This is the piece of information that woke me up to the realization that it was time to put my health back into my own hands. Not that I didn't still need help from health professionals, but that I would become a player in the process of understanding what my options really were and what would be best for me. Here it is: *The vast majority of curricula that are taught in medical schools in this country were put together by organizations that were founded by, or are funded by, pharmaceutical companies.* Read that again.

So let me get this straight... The people who make the most money from our being sick are the same people who are teaching our doctors how to make us healthy? I need you to stop and think about that for just a second with the intelligent part of your brain—not the part that just listens to what we're taught, or to what the media or our friends say, and simply accepts it.

How Medications Work

Before I talk about how medications work, please make sure you understand that in no way am I suggesting you stop taking any medications you are currently using. In most cases, medication is doing a job, and the person taking it needs that medication to continue doing its job, so just chucking it in the trash could be dangerous for some people. But once you begin to understand why you're likely dealing with the issues that you're dealing with, and how some people improve them by making better choices and enabling body chemistry to move in the right direction, then you can decide for yourself if you want to accomplish that. Once you improve an issue by making more ideal decisions, you can then discuss with your doctor the possibility of reducing, or removing, any meds. But promise me you won't try to do this on your own because that's just dumb. If you're currently on any meds, chances are great that you are going to need help from a professional; and the knowledge you receive in this book will be a great starting point to help you make better choices and communicate more effectively with that professional.

Here's how most medications work. Nearly all medications are synthetic, man-made substances; otherwise the manufacturer couldn't patent the drugs and make billions because it's not legal to patent a natural substance. However, most synthetic substances that enter the body will be filtered out by the liver and removed. That's the liver's job. So, if you put a drug in, the liver will filter it out; and the drug won't be able to stay in the body and fulfill its purpose, rendering it worthless. To correct this, manufacturers upped the dosages in drugs to overwhelm the liver so enough of the drug can stay in your system and do the job (or give a physiological reaction) as it is intended to do. Well, guess what? It works. The liver can't remove all of it and the drug often corrects the symptom it was intended to correct. Yet it does so at the cost of punching your liver in the mouth with every dose. Not only can this eventually lead to liver damage (which is why nearly every drug commercial states something along the lines of, "not to be used by those with liver disease"), but even in the first dose the drug is overwhelming the liver and restricting the liver from doing the job it was intended to do: Removing foreign and toxic substances. As the liver gets backed up and can't remove enough junk, the body will often store this junk in fat cells, or deposit it into joints and tissues.

Think of it like that episode of *I Love Lucy* when Lucy is working in the chocolate factory on the conveyor belt. As the chocolate starts to come in faster than she has the ability to keep up, she starts to cram the chocolate in her mouth, pockets, hat, anywhere she can find a safe place. If the body left junk in your bloodstream, it could disrupt the delicate balance and you could literally die. Since the balance of the bloodstream is so important, the body wouldn't let that extreme imbalance happen so it just stores bad stuff in fat cells or other tissues and plans on coming back later to remove it when the coast is clear. Unfortunately, with our taking medications consistently and constantly punching our liver in the mouth, along with all the junk we put in our bodies, the coast is never clear and we can begin to swell like the Stay Puft Marshmallow Man as we accumulate stored water, fat or toxicity in places where it should not be. So, when we gain weight, it is actually our body's way of saving our life. Now, weight gain does have its own health dangers when it becomes excessive, but isn't it smarter for the body to gain weight until the excess weight causes a problem over the choice of dying this Thursday because of all the toxins left in the bloodstream? This is only one possible cause for weight gain. I go over many more possibilities in my book, *Kick Your Fat in the Nuts*. You can also watch video clips from my upcoming documentary, *Why Am I So Fat?*, at www.WhyAmISoFatMovie.com. This film is scheduled for release in early 2018.

Getting The Most From This Book

There are a number of factors that can cause constipation and those reasons truly are different for everyone. To give a high percentage of readers an opportunity to start seeing improvements right away, I have ordered the chapters according to their priority, in my opinion. Each chapter covers a topic, or group of ideas, so that you can move through one chapter at a time and implement what you learn as you go. You may find that some chapters don't apply to you at all. Keep in mind, topics I placed at the beginning of the book are there for a reason. The early chapters cover the problems that need to be addressed in one way or another by most people dealing with constipation.

The final appendix section holds all the advanced, geeky stuff for those who really want to jump into the rabbit hole.

We're all walking around in these bodies that are pretty much the most amazing mechanisms on the planet, yet we hardly know how the human body works. Pharmaceutical companies bombard us with so many ads that we all feel like we're dying before we're thirty. Ads like, "Do you have hair growing out of the top of your head? Have you ever sneezed? Click here to find out if you may be at risk for face cancer." A freaked-out public is a public that spends money in fear. Education about how your body functions can relieve fears.

Testing Tools You'll Need For This Book

In chapter five, I dig in to simple self-testing and how to look at your own chemistry and get a picture of how your body is operating. Before you get to that, I want to touch on some tools that will be helpful so you can get a hold of them before you get to that section of the book. You'll be able to find most of the tools and supplements I talk about in this book at www.NaturalReference.com. The testing tools are also available at just about any drug store and/or health food store in your area. The supplements I use can be harder to access. I had such a hard time finding the supplements that I found to be effective that I partnered with some online retailers to create a store so I could tell them exactly what needed to be made available to the public. Yes, it can be annoying to spend money on tools to improve your health, but at least you don't have to try forty different products like I did to find the ones that do the job. See there, I did some more research for you.

pH Testing Strips

> Some drug stores carry these and most health food stores keep them in stock. Just don't let them sell you other "alkalizing" products when they see you picking up pH testing strips. There is a LOT of bad information out there about pHs, so don't waste your time on that frontier like I did. You'll learn the truth about pHs later in this book. A package or roll of pH strips will usually run between $10-18. Health store clerks also sell a lot of

ketone strips to those on a ketogenic diet so be sure they don't send you home with ketone strips when you ask for pH strips. Avoid buying the type of pH strips with two different colored boxes on the same strip. These strips will often show one reading for one of the colors, and another reading for the second color. pH strips with one testing box or the pH testing tape seems to bring better results. You can see the type that I use at www.NaturalReference.com.

Blood Pressure Cuff

This is a great tool if you're constipated, and one I would recommend buying. The money you spend will be well worth having the ability to monitor your progress. You can get a good one for around $40. Many of you won't know if you're on the right track without one. I like the push-button style that does all the work for you and has a cuff that is easy to put on yourself. It usually does not matter which one you get, as long as you have a way to see if you're improving or if you need to make adjustments. You can also buy the arm wrap in different sizes if needed. The wrist types are okay too, but generally not as accurate and seem to run a little low on the reading. Many drug stores also have those big sit-down machines that allow you to check your blood pressure while you're in the store. These are suitable if a blood pressure cuff is not in your budget, but it sure is nice to be able to check your blood pressure at home when you need to.

Stopwatch

You can also use a common digital kitchen timer or anything with a second hand. Or, I am also pretty sure there is an app for that.

Glucometer

This tool is not always crucial when it comes to improving constipation, but it can provide huge insights into other health factors. A glucometer is actually a great tool to own and every household in the country should have one. The glucometer is sold separately from the glucometer testing strips because the strips expire, whereas the glucometer does not. You can find a glucometer pretty cheap these days, and the strips vary in price from $10 to $40 for a pack of fifty. If you have friends who are diabetic, ask them if you can use their glucometer one morning before you eat anything. If you find that your blood sugar is in a good range, you might be able to go without this tool for a while if you need to budget things out.

Wha'd He Say?

So far, you've learned:

- There is no one remedy that will work for every case of constipation.
- I'm a dork.
- The people that profit the most from us being sick are the same people teaching our doctors how to keep us healthy.
- In order to get the most from this book, you need to acquire a few simple testing tools so you can look at your own chemistry and see how your body is operating.

CHAPTER TWO

Seriously? I Just Wanna Poop!

If you've been constipated for a while now, taking the steps to correct this issue may be one of the best things you ever do for yourself. Once you understand the variety of problems that can create constipation, I have a feeling you're going to be a little upset that nobody has supplied you with the information I'm about to share. I hope you're ready, because it's about to get jazzy.

What's Behind Constipation?

Be mindful that just because an issue *can* create constipation doesn't mean that it is the cause behind *your* constipation. I feel that it is important for you to understand the causes behind the causes. Understanding will make it easier and more motivating to do the work to improve those underlying causes. Answers to your "whys" can also reduce anxiety and remove that "why does this happen to me?" feeling.

An inability to poop is often the result of a combination of circumstances—and that combination can be different for each person. For example, chapter three talks about proper digestion and how this one factor is a very common underlying cause for constipation. However, the reasons that a person may be having digestive issues, or how those issues are manifesting trouble in the body, can be different for each of us.

Some of the topics I cover may be familiar to you. Some you may have instinctively believed to be true. And some will fully freak you out. In any case, know that you may have to re-learn concepts you believed to be true in the past. My question will be, did those concepts work for you? If they did, you would probably be reading a different book right now. Maybe that Tina Fey book? I hear it's funny.

Why Can't I Poop? All My Friends Poop.

Constipation is not socially selective. Each individual has unique chemistry that is likely different from every other person in the world—much like a fingerprint. But if we look at the chemistry of an individual, we can begin to get an idea of what issues may be causing constipation in that individual. That would explain how two friends could literally eat identical foods, yet one friend would have a bowel movement every day while the other friend can make a roll of toilet paper last three weeks.

One person has a body chemistry or functionality that allows him to empty his bowels on a daily basis, while the other friend's body is operating in a manner that prevents that from happening. In my opinion, this is not a curse that you are just stuck with. We all deserve to poop. You deserve to poop.

It's Not About Fiber And Probiotics

If you Google "Fix Constipation," the results you come up with are nothing short of useless. Really? Go for walk? I'm constipated, I didn't twist my ankle playing kickball. I can't simply "walk it off." Fiber and probiotics seem to round up the most frequently seen tips for constipation. Though both fiber and probiotics can be a very small piece of the puzzle for some individuals, they are rarely enough to fix the problem. We will talk more about fiber and probiotics in chapter eight. For now, just know that these two remedies are not the answer. Using fiber to fix constipation is like trying to push a ping pong ball through a metal pipe. It's not going to work.

Once we go over the causes of constipation in the next section, you'll see that drinking more water is the only common advice that has any true merit for constipation. The problem is, depending on your individual body chemistry, drinking more water may simply make you pee more. Or worse, it could cause fatigue, or even depression. Yes, you read that correctly. Even something as "healthy" as drinking more water is not truly right for every person.

Instead of looking at remedies, we're going to look at YOU. When you look at how your body is operating, the reason (or reasons) for YOUR constipation should begin to become more clear.

What Causes The Cork?

There are really only two main causes for constipation, and then a few variables that contribute to the problem. You're about to learn both of those main causes. The rest of the book will be me helping you figure out which of the causes is giving you trouble, and what to do about it.

Major Constipation Cause #1

Stool moves at its level of acidity. In other words, the speed at which your stool moves through your body can be determined by how acidic that stool is. In chapter three I explain digestion and different variables that could cause a stool to be too acidic, or not acidic enough. In any case, if your stool is too alkaline (the opposite of acidic) the alkalinity can reduce the speed at which the stool moves through your intestinal tract, causing you to get backed up. For example, you may have been told that you just have slow motility, or a slow peristalsis response. These are just fancy terms for "your poop doesn't move very quickly." Most doctors will tell you this is caused by genetics or maybe just bad poop luck. You will learn differently in this book.

Major Constipation Cause #2

Stool moves according to the amount of water that is being sent to the bowels. It is possible for a person to be drinking less than enough water. In these cases, a person can simply consume more water and this can often start moving things in the right direction. If you're a person who does not like to drink water, there is usually a reason for that and you will learn how to deal with that in chapter six.

In most cases, however, the lack of water being sent to the bowels is caused by an imbalance in that person's chemistry. When water is being removed from the body, this waste is normally divided between the kidneys and bowels. In chapter five I introduce you to a problem that can occur at the cellular level of your body called an Anabolic Imbalance. If a person is dealing with an Anabolic Imbalance, the body will send more water to the kidneys and less to the bowels. This can cause the stool to become dry, hard, and difficult to move.

An Anabolic Imbalance can also cause a person to pee more often. These individuals will often need to get up and pee in the middle of the night if they are drinking an appropriate amount of water. Urination is more frequent because a larger percentage of the water is being sent to the kidneys. People often think they have to pee so often because they must have a bladder the size of an acorn. Well, I don't know, I've never seen your bladder. But odds are, your body may be simply sending more of your water to your kidneys and less to your bowels. An increase in urination and a decrease in pooping action is a common result.

In chapter five, I teach you how to run simple self-tests to get a better idea of whether or not you're dealing with an Anabolic Imbalance. Before we do that, I cover digestion in chapters three and four. When it comes to constipation, if you need to make improvements to digestion, that will be your priority. Chapter three will help you determine if that's the right move for you.

Water's Role In Constipation

Like I mentioned above, water moving through the bowels is crucial when it comes to improving constipation. However, simply increasing the amount of water you drink may not be enough. Once you learn how to look at your own chemistry in chapter five, you'll start to get a better idea of whether you need to increase your water intake, or simply help your body adjust where most of your water is being sent. You'll also better understand whether or not increasing your water intake could cause problems in other areas. After all, you don't want to improve constipation just to increase depression, sugar cravings, or dizzy spells. In this regard, don't go and pound a gallon of water while you finish this chapter. You may need to fix other issues before you qualify to increase your water intake.

My Mother And Grandmother Were Constipated Too

Pharmaceutical companies love for us to believe that we have been handed down our maladies. "If the issue that you're dealing with is genetic, there's nothing you can do about it and you might as well take this pill we can prescribe to you." The truth is, you can do something about it. It's true that our genes can provide us with a body that tends to lean toward malfunction with more ease. However, most of you reading these words can still move your chemistry and correct issues with nutrition and lifestyle choices. The key word there is "choices."

You have options, and this book gives you the tools you need to make those options work for you. It's going to take effort. Don't think it will be easy. But if you read through this book, your days of thinking that you are hopeless will be over. You may still choose to do nothing about your constipation. Some people aren't interested in putting effort toward their goals. That's okay. Sometimes effort is not that fun. But you will know there are steps you can take to figure out what will work for you, and you will know those options will be here for you when the time is right.

I know I haven't gotten to any of those steps yet, but I'm just too excited. I have to ask... Do you think you're going to be ready to do the work? If you are, it is going to be so fun to hear from you. Maybe you'll post on my Facebook page from the toilet. You can simply say, "Hey Tony, I'm on the toilet and I'm not painting my toenails." Don't think I get tired of hearing success stories. It's the best part of my day, so keep them coming. You know what? If you're a little ballsy, you should tweet to me right now at @kickitinthenuts. Say, "Hey Tony, I'm in chapter two and I'm ready to pop the cork." When you say something out loud, especially where others can see it, it makes the follow-through a whole lot easier. C'mon. Tweet it up.

"You may be born with a genetic map, but that does not mean you have to take the trip."
-Me

I Can Fix This?

Yes, I believe you can fix this. As a matter of fact, I know you can because I've literally heard from hundreds of people who have fixed their constipation using what I teach in this book. And I heard from them before I even wrote this book. Since I teach about digestion in all my books, readers of my weight loss book, or my book on menstrual cramps, or even just listeners to our radio show, *Kick It Naturally*, have all reported improvements to constipation issues. I know you bought this book to improve your constipation, but once you understand how your specific body is operating, don't be surprised if you accidentally improve other issues as well. Remember, most of our books are basically the same book. Each title teaches readers the same steps of how to look at their own body chemistry, and then simply digs deeper into understanding the specific issue the reader is working to improve. But the basics are all the same. Learn how to look at YOU.

To improve the constipation issue, you will simply have the option to figure out what is going wrong, then take steps to improve the underlying cause of that problem. For example, if your self-tests indicate that your body may not be sending enough water to your bowels, you will be able to make adjustments to your nutrition and/or supplementation to help improve that imbalance. If you can improve that imbalance, the body will likely begin sending more water to your bowels and this can loosen up your stool.

If the information you learn in this book leads you to believe that your stool may be leaning too alkaline, you'll be able to take steps to increase the acidity of your stomach contents and help your stool move with more ease. Now, there are tons of variations that can occur with both of the problems I've described here. There are also a wide variety of approaches an individual can take to improve these issues. I take you step by step through this process in this book. I want you to be able to figure out what steps are going to work best for you. Trying remedy after remedy is annoying and usually leads to failure, so let's skip that route. If you follow the steps outlined in this book, you will have a better idea of the approach that will work for you and your body chemistry, before you even get started. It gets fun!

Understanding Digestion Can Help You Tweak Your Digestion

In the following chapter, I teach you about digestion in a way that will make it easier to understand. There are aspects of digestion that may seem a little off topic, but stick with me. There are two main sides to digestion, and it's important to understand them both if you want to poop like a champion. You may also find that you have been dealing with other digestive symptoms that are completely related to your constipation.

If you can understand how digestion is intended to work, and get a better idea of what might not be functioning properly in your body, that will give you the starting point you're looking for. The next two chapters will be the most important chapters in this book.

Working With A Health Coach

Many topics in this book will be very simple, while some will get a little advanced. Keep in mind that there are professional health coaches around the world who understand how to look at your individual body chemistry and provide you with answers that you're looking for. In chapter ten I discuss how to find a professional near you. For now, if at any time you feel overwhelmed, know that help is available.

What To Expect

In this book, you're going to find answers. Answers to questions that you may have had your whole life. Most people who spend their life dealing with discomforts or issues feel like that's just the way it is for them and there's nothing they can do about it. Issues like:

- Cravings
- Skin Issues
- Bloating
- PMS (if you're a menstrual-cycle-type person)
- Weight Gain
- Acid Reflux

The list goes on and on. Guess what? You can do something about it—all of it.

Wha'd He Say?

In this chapter, you learned:
- Instead of looking for a remedy for constipation, this book will teach you how to take steps to correct *your* constipation.
- Stool moves at its level of acidity.

- The amount of water that your body is sending to your bowels can dictate how easily your stool will move.
- The fact that your whole family is constipated doesn't mean that you have to be constipated too.

CHAPTER THREE

Digestion

Everything Goes Back To Digestion

Digestion is a huge deal when it comes to health. It's a shame that the whole digestive process is often swept under the rug. To fix constipation, we really need to look under the rug and better understand how the digestive system works. When I talk about digestion, I'm talking about people's ability to properly break down the foods they are eating. We all tend to assume that if food goes in one end and we have the energy to get out of bed, everything is working as planned. That is not always the case. Digestive issues are actually much more common than you might think. To illustrate: Line up 100 high school boys. You will likely find that the percentage of guys whose pants do not fit properly coincides with the percentage of people in this country who have some type of digestive issue. I know! That's a really high percentage. (And why don't they buy pants that fit... why?)

Diet is what a person eats but nutrition is what the cells see. Nutrition not making it to the cells is where we find the big disconnect. People think that if they focus on foods that are higher in specific nutrients, calcium for example, they're improving their calcium levels with these food choices. Little do they realize, if the body can't properly break down the food they are eating, they're just treating their toilets to calcium-rich poop.

That's what we're doing when we digest. We're breaking down that food into elemental parts that can be used by the body. Believe it or not, the body cannot run on a peanut butter sandwich any more than your car can run on crude oil. It just won't work. However, what the body *can* do is break down that peanut butter sandwich into minerals, amino acids, fats and sugars—and then use those nutrients. Your body needs those nutrients. When digestion is not working properly and you can no longer break down your food enough to pull the required nutrients out of what you have eaten, bodily systems can begin to fail, just like your car would fail if it ran out of gas.

In order for digestion to function properly, there are processes that MUST be in place for most of the nutrients to be pulled from the food you eat. With digestive issues, not only are you missing out on nutrients, but undigested food now becomes a problem that your body has to deal with. If food is not digested, it rots and ferments, which creates gases and toxins. This explains how it doesn't really matter if you're eating organic, extra-virgin, all-natural, grass-fed, hormone-free lima beans washed by the prince of New Guinea. If you can't digest it, it will rot and ferment, creating garbage in your body.

Remember, the methods I explain in this chapter are not magical constipation relief secrets for everyone to implement. If your constipation is not directly caused by digestive malfunctions, following the suggestions in this chapter may not do very much. First, figure out if you need help with your digestion. To give you a benchmark, out of twenty clients who come to me, only one of them will appear to have a properly functioning digestive system. Some readers won't need to follow all the guidelines in this chapter; but if you are experiencing constipation on a regular basis, odds are great that you could do something to improve your digestion.

When looking at an individual, I like to know as much about his or her chemistry as possible. Because this is not always an option, there are questions you can ask to get a good sense of how your body is operating. In chapter five, I add self-tests you can run. Those, coupled with the following questions that you can ask yourself, will allow you to get a great picture of the exact nutritional changes that may benefit you the most.

How's Your Digestion?

In case you failed the last quiz miserably, I'll include a few of the same questions below to give you another chance to get a better score.

(1) Do you frequently pass gas?
        YES NO
(2) Do you often burp after meals or feel bloated? (Even just small burps.)
        YES NO
(3) Does your meal ever feel like it's sitting in your stomach like a rock for too long?
        YES NO
(4) Do you crave sweet or salty foods?
        YES NO
(5) Do some foods make you nauseous?
        YES NO
(6) Is your stool sometimes lighter than the color of corrugated cardboard?
        YES NO
(7) Do you ever experience heartburn or acid reflux?
        YES NO
(8) Have you recently taken any antacids or acid reflux medications?
        YES NO
(9) Are you frequently constipated? Hello?
        YES NO
(10) Do you ever see undigested food in your stool?
        YES NO

If you answered yes for one or more of those questions, you should pay special attention to this chapter.

If you answered yes for two or more of those questions, you will likely need to take action in order to get your digestion back on track.

If you answered yes for three or more of those questions, this chapter will likely change your life.

The Digestive Summary

Digestion is such an important factor when it comes to constipation and a bevy of other health issues, that I've dedicated this entire chapter to explaining the whole system. I even explain strategies you can implement right away to begin to improve your digestion. In that way, by the time you get to chapter six and begin to figure out how whacked your chemistry is, at least you will have already taken steps to improve digestion and you'll be on your way to being a real human. Stand clear because you're going to enter biology class for just a few minutes. I promise to avoid any frog dissecting flashbacks.

When we eat, our stomachs make hydrochloric acid (HCL). This stomach acid, as it is often called, has a pH of around 0.8. The pH scale goes from zero to fourteen. Zero means acidity to the max. Fourteen means alkalinity to the max.

When contents of the stomach (what we eat and drink) are mixed with this stomach acid, that combination will ideally have a pH between 2.0 and 3.0, which is still very acidic. The acidic product created by mixing stomach acid with the food you eat then goes into the duodenum (first ten inches of the small intestine). The other half of the digestive process comes from the bile that is produced by your liver. (I say "half" loosely because there are other factors that contribute to digestion that are not important for this explanation. But for the most part, the main factors in digestion are the acid created in the stomach and the alkaline bile produced by the liver.) Between meals, bile is stored in the gallbladder where it is concentrated up to 18 times. When acid product from the stomach moves into the duodenum, bile from the gallbladder is dropped onto this acid product. In the same way that HCL is acidic, bile is alkaline (which is the opposite of acidic).

Bile meeting stomach acid is like dropping baking soda into vinegar, just like at least one sixth grader does every year when he makes his version of a volcano for his science fair project. In fact, you should try that now. You don't need to build the whole volcano, but you can put a little bowl in your kitchen sink, put a couple teaspoons of baking soda in the bowl, and then slowly pour in a little vinegar. You'll hear a sizzle and see it start to foam up. C'mon, really do it! All the cool kids are doing it. It's a great visualization of what can happen when two substances with opposite pHs meet.

This is the magic of digestion. When the body drops bile onto the contents that comes from the stomach, you get a sizzle, and this is what you're living on. This is what makes everything that was in the food break apart and become available for your body to use. Without this sizzle, foods you eat can't be assimilated. Nutrients and minerals can't be properly extracted and utilized by your body if this action is missing. That's why you hear so many people say, "Health is like a science fair project." Okay, I've never heard anyone say that; but if you don't have that sizzle in your digestion, you might as well be that 12-year-old holding the volcano with an "F" on it because the damn lava didn't come out. You've got to have the sizzle.

If there isn't enough stomach acid, there won't be that sizzle. If there isn't enough bile to drop down onto the food that was mixed with the stomach acid, there won't be that sizzle. In order for digestion to work properly, every step of that process has to be active. Otherwise, instead of a sizzle, you get more of a fizzle; and you may break down just a very small portion of your food, or your food will partially break down by processes of rotting and fermenting. This rotting and fermenting creates chemical reactions and gases that can cause bloating, burping, nausea, bad breath, upset stomach, and all kinds of other non-fun stuff. Have you ever been around someone who had breath that smelled like a garbage can? Most people look at bad breath as a dental hygiene issue, and it can be; but more often than not it's a situation of, "I have food rotting in my stomach and intestines and the stench it creates is coming out of my mouth." Yes, I know you've met that guy.

This repulsive rotting of last night's dinner can also be the reason you don't feel like eating the next morning. Many of you who always skip breakfast truly have no appetite when you wake up. Some people are even nauseous because last night's dinner still hasn't fully digested and is becoming toxic. Their bodies are telling them, "Look, I haven't finished dealing with last night's food that has now turned into garbage. Please don't dump anything else on top of it." By improving digestion, your morning appetite can also improve.

Give Me Acid Or Give Me Death

A bit of a drama queen? Maybe. Maybe not. A lack of stomach acid can be a huge health concern that can result in even bigger health concerns.

Here are a few of the issues that can come from a need for more stomach acid. I explain some of these further in chapter four when I cover elimination.

- Nutritional deficiency. Almost every nutritional deficiency stems from a lack of stomach acid or a lack of bile flow or poor food selection.

- Burping or bloating. Bloating is almost always due to a lack of stomach acid.
- Frequent stomach discomfort after eating.
- Acid reflux or heartburn. Yes, reflux is usually caused by NOT ENOUGH acid, not too much acid like you see in advertisements. It's one of the biggest health mistakes being made by millions of people today.
- Chronic constipation. I explain the Anabolic Imbalance (that can often contribute to constipation) in detail in chapter six; but a lack of stomach acid is often a factor, if not the main cause, for constipation.
- The door is open for bad critters to sneak into your body. Stomach acid is the barrier that blocks harmful organisms from entering into and through the digestive tract.

Improving Your Stomach Acid

If you need to improve your stomach acid, there are supplements you can use to boost your body's ability to correct these functions. But, before I teach you how to use Betaine HCL supplements to recover your proper stomach acid function, I need to give you a huge flippin' WARNING. READ IT! DON'T IGNORE IT!!!!

*** HCL Warning ***

If you're going to use HCL, be sure to also use Beet Flow (explained below in *You Need Good Bile Flow*) or a similar product. I never allow any of my clients to use HCL unless they are also using Beet Flow. If you don't have your bile flowing correctly and you add more acid into the stomach, you could create a duodenal ulcer or other issues. I cover all of this in more detail in chapter four. I just want to make sure you understand not to use HCL without also using Beet Flow. It is also imperative to read *How to Use HCL Supplements* below before you begin supplementing with HCL.

Why Use HCL

We all know the body makes stomach acid. But when we hear about stomach acid, it's usually how people have "too much" acid and that's why they are dealing with heartburn or acid reflux issues. There is a lot of brilliant marketing by the pharmaceutical companies when it comes to stomach acid and why it might be a good idea to turn acid off, and I believe it the same way I believe that a mime is a talented artist. In

Appendix A, I explain why people really get heartburn and reflux, but let's first look at why "turning off" your stomach acid with drugs is one of the worst possible things you can do for your long-term health.

Hydrochloric acid (HCL) is the protector of the human body. Let's say you are eating at the buffet and you're taking in viruses, bacteria, and microorganisms because you scoop up the salad the kids sneezed on a few minutes earlier. While you eat from this salad bar, you are taking in all this filth and you are eating undercooked hamburger and chicken drumettes that were dropped on the floor. The truth is you don't really know what you are getting. Keep in mind that I worked at a salad bar when I was a kid, and my only rule was that being funny in front of the cute waitresses was far more important to me than delivering clean, sanitary food to all the redneck patrons that came in on coupon night. Your food doesn't even need to be dropped on the floor by a zit-faced high school kid to have bacteria or other little creatures on it. Even the food you clean and prepare at home can have some little ninja-like varmints that make it through the cleaning process. (Varmints! 500 points to me for fitting in a Yosemite Sam reference.)

That's where HCL becomes such a hero. Anything that comes into YOU (any microorganisms, bacteria, or other types of bad guys) is going to die in an acid bath. That stomach acid is the protector of the mechanism that is YOU. The hydrochloric acid function of the stomach is your knight in very disgusting armor. When you take a drug that turns that barrier off, you're opening the door to anybody that wants to come in and raid the pantry (you are the pantry in this scenario). That's why two people can eat the same meal and one will get food poisoning and have projectile fluids coming out of both ends, and the other person will just say, "The fish didn't taste right, did it? Oh, and sorry about your luck." One person had the proper level of stomach acid to kill whatever little bastards were still living on that fish; and the other person is praying to the porcelain god, vowing to never eat seafood again.

The point is, you want that acid function to be in the stomach because it is the gatekeeper. It's the lock that keeps all the hoodlums out. I don't want you to think that taking medication for acid reflux or heartburn is the only reason a person may lose that acid function. There are many ways a person can produce less than the proper levels of acid. There are also many reasons the acid function may not fully recover for years, or even decades.

The body needs minerals in order to generate stomach acid. However, the body needs stomach acid in order to fully break down foods and pull minerals out of those foods. Without digestion, you can't assimilate minerals, but without minerals, you can't create proper digestion. See how someone could be screwed with a capital "F" for a long time? Using HCL supplementation can allow you to manufacture proper digestion so you can pull the minerals out of the food you are eating. Once the body has enough minerals, the stomach can often begin to make an appropriate amount of HCL. At this point, the HCL supplementation can often be reduced until the body is making plenty of its own HCL—and then the supplementation can be removed altogether. Depending on your mineral reserves, food choices, and many other factors, this process can take weeks, months, or longer. However, it often doesn't take a long time to begin to feel like you're improving. In any case, a stool that is more acidic will often move more easily and progress through the system at a faster pace. As you can see, improving subpar stomach acid levels is often a big piece of the constipation puzzle.

How to Use HCL Supplements

Hydrochloric Acid (HCL), also labeled as Betaine HCL, is the most widely needed digestive supplement in my opinion. It's also the one that comes with the most important instructions. This is NOT a supplement you want to take willy-nilly. (Isn't it amazing that such a ridiculous phrase like "willy-nilly" could become so widely accepted? That bugs me.) Here is a list of important guidelines to follow while using HCL supplements:

- HCL capsules should always be taken in the middle of the meal and chased by at least one bite of food. If the capsules were to get stuck in your esophagus and dissolve there, it could feel like heartburn.
- Start by taking one capsule with a meal containing no starches. This means avoid foods like potatoes, bread, pasta, cereal, rice, etc. If you don't feel any new digestive discomfort after the meal, and your stool does not become too loose, you know it's okay to move up to two capsules at your next meal. You can continue in this manner until you reach a maximum of five capsules per meal. Once you reach the full dose of five capsules per meal, most people can add a few

starches back into their diet without experiencing any reflux or heartburn symptoms.
- Most people will hold at five capsules per meal for months. So, if your digestive symptoms disappear, it may be time to begin reducing your dose. The goal is to see if your body has started making more of its own HCL, reducing your need to supplement with capsules. At your next meal, you can reduce by one capsule and hold at that dose for a few days to make sure none of your digestive symptoms come back. You can continue to reduce your dose in this manner until you no longer need to take any HCL capsules. If you lower your dose to one or two capsules per meal, and symptoms return, you know you may need to use a higher dose for a while longer. The most helpful signs to watch, when determining proper stomach acidification are: burping, bloating, constipation, acid reflux, heartburn, seeing food in your stool, or discomfort after eating (especially if you feel like your food is just sitting in your stomach like a rock). Any of these symptoms are possible indications that your food is not yet being properly acidified.
- If your stomach becomes extremely uncomfortable when you begin HCL supplementation, yet you know you experience symptoms that often indicate a lack of stomach acid, you may be dealing with a bacterial infection in your stomach. If bacteria have set up camp in your stomach (which is extremely common when the stomach is not creating enough HCL), the waste from that bacteria could be making the stomach even more alkaline. When dumping HCL into a highly alkaline environment, the reaction between the acid and alkaline substances can create a fizzy mess. That interaction can create gasses and cause pressure and make you feel very uncomfortable. If this is the case for you, you may need to take steps to wipe out a layer of that bacteria before you can begin to implement HCL. I cover how to reduce bacteria in the stomach in chapter ten when I talk about d-limonene and a few more supplements that can be helpful for some individuals.
- Be sure to adjust your dose according to the amount of protein in each meal. If you have a meal with very little protein, you may need to reduce the number of capsules you use with that meal. I don't suggest using HCL supplementation if you're only having a protein shake.
- If you experience any diarrhea or loose stool issues after you begin to use HCL, reduce what you are taking until you can improve your bile flow using the suggestions found below in *Improving Your Bile Flow*. If you have more acid than your bile flow can handle, that can create a loose stool issue. This may not mean that you don't need the acid, you may just need to improve your bile flow before you can handle more acid. If you

experience this issue, read more about loose stool issues in chapter four.
- If you experience magnified acid reflux when you begin using HCL, be sure to read about Acid Reflux in Appendix A so you know what steps to take to correct this. Occasionally, an individual who has never experienced acid reflux will feel heartburn symptoms when first starting HCL. Appendix A explains how this is almost always caused by not having ENOUGH acid. These symptoms will normally stop once your stomach is acidic enough to trigger your LES valve to close so food can't reflux up your esophagus. I go over this in much more detail in Appendix A.

You Need Good Bile Flow

Bile is what allows us to emulsify the fats we eat so they can be used by the body. All food is either carbohydrate, protein or fat. To process the fats, you need bile. Bile is not only needed for proper digestion, bile is also the main exit pathway for filth and toxins from the body. Junk that can't be removed can often get stored in fat cells, so this is a huge factor. Here are a few of the issues that can come from a need for improved bile flow.

- Nutritional deficiency. Almost every nutritional deficiency stems from either a lack of stomach acid or a lack of bile flow. Poor food selection is usually the third factor.
- Passing gas. It can be a big indication that bile is not flowing correctly.
- Weight gain.
- Chronic diarrhea or issues like colitis, crohns, IBS, etc.
- Duodenal ulcer.
- Chronic acne.
- Stool color that is sometimes lighter than corrugated cardboard.

Improving Your Bile Flow

In chapter six I talk about an imbalance that can cause your bile to become too thick and sticky and encumber its ability to flow correctly. For most people, however, using a supplement made predominantly of beet greens is enough to correct the problem. Beet greens have an amazing ability to help thin the bile so it will flow properly. Unfortunately, you would likely need to eat an entire bucket of beet tops on a daily basis in order to get the effect you're looking for. A concentrated supplement is far more effective and will allow you to avoid eating meals fit for a horse.

There are many beet supplements out there, but few contain as much of the organic beet green as Beet Flow from Empirical Labs. This is the one I use with my clients. It is absolutely the most expensive supplement I use, but it's well worth the money. If you are willing to do the work to correct digestion, this upgrade could help improve any number of ailments you are dealing with, reducing the number of remedies you may buy in an attempt to fix your woes. In this regard, investing in Beet Flow can turn out to actually save you money.

Why Use Beet Flow

If you're going to use HCL, you need to use Beet Flow as well. You really need to make sure your bile is flowing correctly if you're going to be adding more acid to your stomach. That acid needs to be neutralized by bile when it reaches the duodenum. If you want to digest your food correctly, you need both sides of digestion working properly.

How to Use Beet Flow

Most people use only two or three capsules per meal. You can take them before or during your meal.

Note: If you are on birth control medication, be sure to read about it in Appendix A. It will freak you out. Birth control medication has the ability to thicken the bile, reducing its ability to flow properly.

Add Digestive Enzymes

Enzymes are another factor of the digestive process. All living foods are meant to contain enzymes that actually help you digest that food better. Yet, with today's despicable farming methods, even many raw foods do not contain the needed enzymes to correctly digest those foods. On top of that, any time food is processed or heated over 118 degrees (pretty much any time you cook food), the enzymes are killed and you will not get the full benefit from that food. In order to fully break down the food you eat, you can supplement enzymes with your food. As we age, the body's stockpile of usable enzymes diminishes. People over thirty should be supplementing enzymes with their food. If you don't supply your body with the enzymes it needs, your body steals enzymes intended for repair processes and turns them into digestive enzymes, leaving fewer repair-enzymes for their intended use.

Enzymes facilitate a food's ability to break down and mix with water. In an effort to increase shelf-life, much of today's produce has been modified to depress enzymes contained within those foods. Using digestive enzymes can help overcome this problem.

With certain imbalances, TOO MANY enzymes can facilitate deterioration. So, you want to take just enough to help you digest your food. Many enzyme companies promote taking unlimited enzymes but that is not recommended with certain imbalances.

How to Use Digestive Enzymes

Most people see improvement by using only one or two capsules per meal.

Where To Get Supplements

The beginning of chapter ten covers the world that is consumer supplement sales. There is a reason you hear so much good and bad about supplement use. Supplements are good only if you use the right ones for the imbalances you are dealing with, and they are good only if you use high quality products that can be properly absorbed. With many supplements, only a very small percentage of what is in them can be absorbed by the person using them.

I'm not saying that the supplements I recommend are the only good supplements out there. They have simply brought the best results, in my experience. Consumers miss out sometimes since most high-quality companies sell only through practitioners. Empirical Labs is a company that sells most of their products only through qualified professionals. Having a wider variety of quality supplements available to you can be another perk of working with a professional health coach. However, some of Empirical Lab's products are available to consumers as well, since these particular supplements are considered to be safe for people to use, no matter what their chemistry is (so long as they take the time to learn about these products and use a little common sense). This is the brand I implement most frequently for my own use.

Most health food stores sell some form of HCL. I just don't like a lot of them because they contain pepsin and other ingredients that can bother people's stomachs when they start to use more than one capsule per meal. I try to use straight HCL. Also, the capsules I use are 515mg; so if you get something different, be sure to adjust your number of capsules accordingly. I use HCL from Empirical Labs, which can be found on www.NaturalReference.com. This is the only site approved to sell Empirical Lab's products to the public. Beet Flow and the digestive enzyme I prefer, Digesti-zyme, can also be found on this website.

I like the enzyme Digesti-zyme because it contains cofactors, like zinc, that the body can use to make its own HCL. In this regard, Digesti-zyme can reduce how long you may need to supplement HCL.

Supplements Review

www.NaturalReference.com
Brand: Empirical Labs

Betaine HCL (See the HCL warning under *Improving Your Stomach Acid* in this chapter.)
1-5 per meal (In the middle of the meal.)

Beet Flow
2-3 per meal

Digesti-zyme
1-2 per meal

In chapter ten I go over other supplements that can be used for other imbalances. With many of those supplements, I am not as picky about the brand I use with my clients. But when it comes to correcting digestion, I haven't seen anything else work as well as these three.

Wha'd He Say?

In this chapter, you learned:
- When trying to improve constipation, digestion is often a big piece of that puzzle.

- Both sides of digestion are equally important. You must have enough HCL production and you must have proper bile flow.
- Few people with digestive issues are able to truly improve digestion without the temporary aid of supplements.
- Most people will benefit from the use of digestive enzymes.
- You can order Beet Flow, HCL and digestive enzymes from www.NaturalReference.com.

Chapter Four

Elimination & Digestion Gone Wild

Let's Talk Poop

There are two types of people in this world. There are stargazers and there are stoolgazers, and the stoolgazers fare better. There is a lot that can be learned from poop—specifically, how our bodies are operating and, especially, how well digestion is working. Just by buying this book, you already know digestion is not working as planned due to the fact that nothing is coming out the back door.

Better understanding the signs of digestive trouble can guide your efforts toward improving many issues. To better understand why a person may get plugged up, I will also provide a quick explanation of how chronic diarrhea issues can develop. If you know someone who is dealing with Crohn's, Colitis, or IBS, be sure to read about these topics in more detail in Appendix A. We all know that we poop to eliminate waste from the body. Many don't know, however, that stool often moves at its level of acidity, as I explained in chapter two. Stool can move too quickly and be too loose when it is too acidic. Not only does this burn the intestines, but also, if the stool is moving too quickly, the body doesn't get the opportunity to absorb as many nutrients as it should. If stool is not acidic enough, it can move too slowly and can lead to constipation.

If a lack of stomach acid results in stool that is too alkaline and moving too slowly, that waste that was supposed to be removed out the back door (your butt) can get held up in the system too long. If waste is not removed properly, it can be re-absorbed through the intestinal walls and will need to be filtered out all over again. I explain how this can affect the liver later in this chapter. Increasing your stomach acid by supplementing HCL can be a great first step toward improving constipation.

Burping, Bloating And Passing Gas

Keeping an eye on whether you are burping or bloating is one way to get an idea of how acidic your stomach environment is during the digestive process. To figure out if you're really bloating, here's the ultimate question. (This question works only for women because men are way too oblivious of their bodies to get this one.) Are your clothes tighter in the evening when you take them off than in the morning when you put them on? If you so much as have to think about it, you're probably not bloating, because a woman knows. She will say, "Yeah, they are tighter when I take them off." She knows, and if they are tighter, she is bloating. If the acid product in the stomach is not sufficient then people are going to grow bacteria in their tummies. When they grow bacteria in their tummies, they are going to produce gas. It is the same as making beer, wine, champagne or root beer; all of these things are fermented. When you ferment, you are going to get gas and the gas is going to bloat. Some people may feel very bloated, while others may experience more burping.

When I say burping, I don't mean these huge belches. I'm talking about those little burps that are hardly even noticed. Those little burps are usually a good sign that the stomach is not acidic enough. I see a lot of people who don't even realize that they're burping after their meals. Once I ask them, they come back later and say, "Hey, ya know what, I am burping after my meals and I never even noticed." Now, it's your turn to pay attention and see if you're burping too. You may be burping because of the gas created by undigested food rotting and fermenting, or because of the gases created by bacteria that are living in your stomach, or because of a combination of both. Taking stock of what is going on with your body is the first step to making improvements.

People think, "Everyone passes gas, what's the big deal?" The problem is most adults don't have their digestion working correctly anymore and that is why gas is so common. If you're passing gas, it's usually because your bile isn't flowing well enough. If your bile isn't dropping into the duodenum to meet the acid product from the stomach, you're not digesting properly.

Helping Your Liver

I include some thoughts about liver function in this elimination chapter because proper bile flow is such a vital part of how effectively your liver is taking care of business. I say this a lot, and I'll probably say it three or four more times in this book: In my opinion, the two most important factors for good health are digestion and liver function. I'm not trying to say that if people have a horrific imbalance in need of attention, or an extra limb growing out of the side of their head, that they first need to correct liver function. I'm just speaking generally when I say that the liver's ability to handle its affairs is a super big deal.

I've covered a multitude of factors that can reduce a liver's performance: Almost any medication, a lack of bile flow, bringing in more junk than the liver can remove, etc. Any of these things can trouble a liver; and if the liver isn't working optimally, eventually your body won't be working optimally either. Think of your liver like a huge ventilation fan that can clear smoke out of a kitchen or entire house. Growing up as a kid, my family lived in a big yellow two-story house. In the living room, just outside of the bathroom, was a huge ventilation fan that was built into the ceiling.

My Mom had a friend who would come over to the house and smoke in the living room. Even at twelve years old, I hated cigarette smoke and didn't want to smell it in my house any more than I wanted to miss an episode of *The Muppet Show*. Whenever my Mom's friend, Margaret, was over for a visit, I would turn on this huge fan and immediately it would suck all the smoke out of the house, as if it never existed. It's not that the house wasn't big enough to hold Margaret and myself at the same time, it was just too disgusting when that fan wasn't on.

This is similar to how your liver works. To say that your body can't handle a few toxins coming in is far from true. The liver is your body's massive ventilation fan. As junk comes in, the liver moves it out to keep the system clean and operating smoothly. I came home from school one day in a thunderstorm to find that our electricity was out. There was Margaret sitting on the couch. I could barely make out her beady little eyes through all the smoke, but I knew it was her. I immediately turned around to leave the house and my Mom asked where I was going. "Out to get struck by lightning," I said. I guess I was a jackass when I was a kid too. In the same way I was too miserable to exist in that house without the fan, you might be too miserable in your life without your liver working properly.

After all the medical doctors had their way with me, and my liver was trashed from all the drugs I was taking, it was tough to even walk by some substances, much less take them into my body. When the liver is overwhelmed and can't handle the current load that it's already dealing with, it can be arduous for people to find foods they can eat without feeling miserable. There were only three or four very clean foods I could eat without feeling horrible because my body couldn't deal with the chemicals and preservatives found in most foods. Now that I have improved my liver function, those things don't bother me because my body can handle the trouble and my liver can remove those substances.
BIG NOTE: If you have had your gallbladder removed, this can turn into a real problem. Good bile flow is required for proper liver function, and a gallbladder is required for good bile flow. If you've had your gallbladder yanked, be sure to read about gallbladder removal in Appendix A.

Is Constipation Making Me Gain Weight?

As I said, when the liver is overwhelmed and can't remove enough toxicity from the body, the body can store junk in fat cells. This is sort of an emergency back-up plan to take a substance that is harmful and could wreak havoc on the body, and make that substance inert by shoving the toxic stuff into a fat cell. If it is stored in a fat cell, it won't pose any immediate threat. If the body didn't store this junk in fat cells, these toxins could upset the delicate balance of the bloodstream and we could literally die. In that regard, thank you, fat. Thank you for helping me avoid death today.

When an individual is constipated and waste is not being removed out the back door, that lingering waste can increase the toxic load the liver has to deal with. As this waste is reabsorbed into the bloodstream through the intestinal walls, the body starts to say, "Hey, I already sent this garbage out of here." As more and more toxins get stored in fat cells, yes, in a roundabout way, constipation can easily lead to weight gain.

Before we wrap up this chapter, I want to explain more issues that can cause the foods we eat to turn into a problem for us. If there are underlying causes creating constipation, those same underlying causes may be creating much more trouble than you think. If a lack of stomach acid is one of the contributing factors for your constipation, it may also be important to understand food sensitivities.

Conquering Our Food - Food Allergies and Sensitivities

When you eat a salami sandwich (and no, I'm not recommending that you eat a salami sandwich... it's just fun to say salami sandwich), the goal is to conquer that sandwich instead of having it cause all kinds of trouble and carry you off captive. Food allergies are a very hot topic these days; and people come to me all the time and tell me about the testing they had done for food allergies. They tell me their tests showed they're allergic to nuts, dairy, wheat, gluten, soy, pork, turkey jerky, the board game Parcheesi, and Lou Diamond Phillips. Well, at what point does this person have to leave Earth in order to eat lunch? He's been told that he's allergic to just about everything on the planet. If you get to the point where you can eat only things that resemble Al Roker, it might be time to understand food allergies.

You may have already come across some of the rules or diets to help those with food sensitivities. There are gluten-free diets, blood-type diets, food-combining diets, raw-food diets—this list could keep going all the way down to the "*Saved by the Bell*, Zack & Kelly" diet. Most of these diets can actually benefit some individuals, but many people who need to employ a diet like this in order to feel better could find similar relief by correcting any digestive issues. Once you can fully digest what you're eating, the need to complete the "Screech-free" phase of the Zack & Kelly diet becomes obsolete.

So, what are all of these theories about food based on? There are so many books and diets and "gurus" out there it's enough to make you lose your appetite, even if you did know what you were supposed to eat. So, who's right? Do I eat for my blood type? Do I alkalize? Do I avoid carbs? Do I eat whatever I want as long as it starts with the letter "B"? Who's right? Well, I don't know. Whose research was everybody using as a basis for fact when they came up with these diets? Maybe most of the test subjects they used did, indeed, thrive on the ice cream sandwich diet. But, if you're interested in how the human body works, which I know I am, you first need to know how that particular human's digestion is functioning. If digestion is not so great, there is no diet that will fix all that person's woes.

Improper digestion is the reason juicing and blending have become so popular. Many fancy-pants gurus advocate buying these blenders that cost as much as a car and can liquefy your iPhone in thirty seconds. They tell us that we need to liquefy our food or we can't pull the nutrients out. And they're right, if you're a person with horrible digestion. That's why so many people feel better when they start to juice—they're actually getting some nutrients into the system. I do find that these juicing maniacs get a little upset when they learn that simply fixing their digestion can give them the same benefit. "You mean it was unnecessary for me to blend my turkey meatloaf and brussels sprouts and drink it through a straw?"

Let me get back to the point and break down these food allergies a little bit. Enzymes can play a factor in food sensitivities. If people don't have the correct enzymes to break down a specific type of food, that food can give them trouble. Take dairy for example. Many cases of lactose intolerance are just situations where people are lacking the enzyme lactase. If they supplement this enzyme, they may see improvement with their intolerance. The Digesti-zyme supplement I mentioned in chapter three is a broad-based enzyme that includes lactase. However, some individuals will need a supplement with a higher dose of lactase, like Milk-Gest.

The main cause for food allergies, however, normally has more to do with improper digestion than a lack of enzymes. In chapter three, I talked about how your body can't use a peanut butter sandwich until that sandwich has been broken down into elemental nutrients. This same understanding is used when looking at food allergies. Once you break down that peanut butter sandwich, it's no longer a peanut butter sandwich. Instead, it is now minerals, fats, amino acids—the things your body needs and recognizes as nutrients that can be used to rebuild your body.

However, if you never break down that peanut butter sandwich because your digestion is not working properly, that food still has its own identity since it was never conquered. That identity says, "Hi, I'm a peanut butter sandwich." Well, there is no use for a "peanut butter sandwich" in the body. The body can use only the nutrients that are pulled out of that peanut butter sandwich once it has been broken down by a functioning digestive system. If this peanut butter sandwich enters the system absorbed by the bloodstream etc. and still has its own identity, it is looked upon by the body as an invader and will be attacked and removed. A peanut butter sandwich is not going to be recognized as something that can be used. For this reason, the defense system is going to run and scream and sound the alarms. As your immune system creates antibodies to deal with this invader, an imprint of those antibodies is saved in the "security files." Now, the next time you eat a peanut butter sandwich, all hell breaks loose as the system comes down hard on this "invader" and you can feel an "allergic response." And why wouldn't you? Your body just went to war against a peanut butter sandwich for cryin' out loud. You're not supposed to be trying to digest a peanut butter sandwich in your bloodstream using your immune system. **PLEASE NOTE: This is not to say that someone with a peanut allergy or something as severe and life-threatening as that should not take it seriously.** They absolutely should. That is not what I'm talking about here. Most of those individuals were born with an allergy like that. I'm talking about sensitivities that people have developed in their life due to an inability to digest, or conquer, their food.

To better understand steps that may help you improve food sensitivity issues, read chapter nine from my book, *Kick Your Fat in the Nuts*. You can read this entire chapter on my website for free by going to www.KickItNaturally.com and searching for "Remove The Trouble."

Acid Reflux, GERD, & Heartburn

Acid reflux, GERD, and heartburn are all issues that normally arise from digestive issues. If you deal with any of these problems, be sure to read about them in Appendix A now. I promise chapter five will still be there waiting when you come back.

Wha'd He Say?

In this chapter, you learned:
- Become a stoolgazer to gain valuable information about how your digestion is functioning.
- Constipation is often an indication of other problems.
- Increasing bile flow can help your liver clean out more junk, so the junk doesn't get stored in fat cells.

Chapter Five

Simple Self-Testing

You're about to learn how to run very simple physiological tests on your body. The information you gain from these tests will direct you to nutritional choices and lifestyle changes that could help you improve your constipation for the long haul. However, I'm going to share only the simple tests here. If you find that you would like to run additional tests and gain even more information, you can follow the intermediate self-testing instructions in Appendix B. Most readers will learn enough through the simple self-tests to improve their constipation issues. However, if you're also dealing with other health issues, the more advanced tests in Appendix B may be a big help.

This Is The Magic

You have an opportunity here to begin understanding how your specific body is operating. You may be able to recognize imbalances that you are experiencing and you may even find food, nutrition or lifestyle changes that could help improve those imbalances. Just be sure to understand that the body is very complicated. In most cases, if a person is serious about improving a severe symptom, condition, or something even more serious, that individual is going to need help from a professional who has a firm grasp on these foundational principles. So, don't try to be a hero and figure it all out yourself. There really is no reason to show off in that way, and you will likely create added frustration for yourself. I'm going to teach you what to look at and where you can find tools to chart your progress and monitor your changes on your own. I'm also going to show you where you can find help when you need it. Be sure you understand how much time and effort you will save by finding a professional to help you along.

It's important to understand that people need to take responsibility for their own health. Most people will not be able to simply take a few supplements, or remove a few foods from their diet, and correct every issue that may have been developing for the last two or three decades. You will, however, be able to watch your chemistry and see if you are moving in the right direction, even before you might notice any changes in how you feel. For many, improved chemistry is often enough to keep them on track long enough to reap the rewards.

This approach is much different from only treating a symptom. The medical world is not the only place where practitioners treat off of symptom. Most natural practitioners work off of symptoms as well. They just use natural substances to improve those symptoms instead of drugs, but they are still pigeonholing a client into a "diagnosis" based on the symptoms. When working in this manner, a practitioner might as well be asking the clients to throw darts at a "diagnosis dart board." At least with this option, clients might leave the doctor's office with a stuffed animal.

However, when natural practitioners do guess correctly, a natural approach often doesn't bring about an immediate "drug-like" response. Therefore, the client stops or moves on to the next big thing.

When looking to help your body correct its own issues, keep in mind that this process will take much longer than the 4-6 hours it often takes for a drug to kick in. In nature, things that happen fast are often bad things. The best things happen slowly. A flower doesn't wake up and go, "BAM!!!" open. The flower opens very slowly and gradually. The sun doesn't just appear out of nowhere in full force. That would freak us out every single time. The sun rises gradually, just as it sets, just as the grass grows and the seasons change. Let your body do the same. If you're looking to "fix" a problem by Friday because you don't want it to interfere with the big square dance you hope to attend, you're going to find yourself very frustrated—not only because you really need a better social life if a square dance is your big event, but also because you're setting yourself up for failure if you believe you can change the agriculture of your body in a few days. You can't.

Data Tracking Sheet

In this section you will find a *Data Tracking Sheet*. You can also go to the site, www.KickItNaturally.com and download a free PDF to print so you won't have to mark up your pretty book. This will allow you to keep a binder of your progress so you can track your results and see patterns. You will also have that information available in case you decide to seek help from a professional. Click on the link BOOK TOOLS to download the *Data Tracking Sheet*. While you're at it, you can also download the *Basic Imbalance Guide*, as I cover that form in chapter six.

On the top right corner of the *Data Tracking Sheet*, you will see colored boxes that are used when testing your urine with an 11-parameter strip. These strips are used as part of the intermediate testing procedures outlined in Appendix B. You won't need to use those colored boxes unless you decide you want to collect more information about your chemistry.

URINE TEST STRIP
BLOOD Hemolyzed
Non-hemolyzed
UROBILINOGEN
BILIRUBIN
PROTEIN
NITRITE
KETONES
ASCORBIC ACID
GLUCOSE
PH
SPECIFIC GRAVITY
LEUKOCYTES

Date____ Time____	Date____ Time____	Date____ Time____	Date____ Time____
Well-Being_____	Well-Being_____	Well-Being_____	Well-Being_____
Urine pH ____	Urine pH ____	Urine pH ____	Urine pH ____
Saliva pH ____	Saliva pH ____	Saliva pH ____	Saliva pH ____
Breath Rate ____	Breath Rate ____	Breath Rate ____	Breath Rate ____
Breat Hold ____	Breat Hold ____	Breat Hold ____	Breat Hold ____
Resting Standing	Resting Standing	Resting Standing	Resting Standing
Blood Pressure (Systolic) ____ ____	Blood Pressure (Systolic) ____ ____	Blood Pressure (Systolic) ____ ____	Blood Pressure (Systolic) ____ ____
Blood Pressure (Diastolic) ____ ____	Blood Pressure (Diastolic) ____ ____	Blood Pressure (Diastolic) ____ ____	Blood Pressure (Diastolic) ____ ____
Pulse ____ ____	Pulse ____ ____	Pulse ____ ____	Pulse ____ ____

Date____ Time____	Date____ Time____	Date____ Time____	Date____ Time____
Well-Being_____	Well-Being_____	Well-Being_____	Well-Being_____
Urine pH ____	Urine pH ____	Urine pH ____	Urine pH ____
Saliva pH ____	Saliva pH ____	Saliva pH ____	Saliva pH ____
Breath Rate ____	Breath Rate ____	Breath Rate ____	Breath Rate ____
Breat Hold ____	Breat Hold ____	Breat Hold ____	Breat Hold ____
Resting Standing	Resting Standing	Resting Standing	Resting Standing
Blood Pressure (Systolic) ____ ____	Blood Pressure (Systolic) ____ ____	Blood Pressure (Systolic) ____ ____	Blood Pressure (Systolic) ____ ____
Blood Pressure (Diastolic) ____ ____	Blood Pressure (Diastolic) ____ ____	Blood Pressure (Diastolic) ____ ____	Blood Pressure (Diastolic) ____ ____
Pulse ____ ____	Pulse ____ ____	Pulse ____ ____	Pulse ____ ____

Date____ Time____	Date____ Time____	Date____ Time____	Date____ Time____
Well-Being_____	Well-Being_____	Well-Being_____	Well-Being_____
Urine pH ____	Urine pH ____	Urine pH ____	Urine pH ____
Saliva pH ____	Saliva pH ____	Saliva pH ____	Saliva pH ____
Breath Rate ____	Breath Rate ____	Breath Rate ____	Breath Rate ____
Breat Hold ____	Breat Hold ____	Breat Hold ____	Breat Hold ____
Resting Standing	Resting Standing	Resting Standing	Resting Standing
Blood Pressure (Systolic) ____ ____	Blood Pressure (Systolic) ____ ____	Blood Pressure (Systolic) ____ ____	Blood Pressure (Systolic) ____ ____
Blood Pressure (Diastolic) ____ ____	Blood Pressure (Diastolic) ____ ____	Blood Pressure (Diastolic) ____ ____	Blood Pressure (Diastolic) ____ ____
Pulse ____ ____	Pulse ____ ____	Pulse ____ ____	Pulse ____ ____

The Coalition

There is an international association called *The Coalition for Health Education*. This private, nonprofit association spans the planet and consists of doctors, health coaches, nutritionists, a wide variety of other types of natural health professionals and members of the general public who want to learn more about natural health and how the body really works. When readers come to www.KickItNaturally.com looking for a health coach who can help them better understand the ideas that are taught in this book, we send them to *The Coalition* to find a professional in their area.

We have also made arrangements with this private association to allow our readers to become members without sponsorship from a professional health coach. *The Coalition* has an advanced website that was put in place to help health coaches educate their clients and monitor the progress of their clients' chemistry. As those clients input the numbers from their self-tests into the website, the health coach can help them make nutritional adjustments according to their chemistry. However, even if you are not working with a health coach, as one of my readers, you can register as a member of the site, which will grant you access to all of your own advanced monitoring and tracking tools. I helped *the Coalition* put together many of the systems they use today so they have given my readers the hook-up. As you input the results of your self-tests into the system, you can watch the changes over time in the site's dynamic graphing systems. You can even keep a food journal to which your self-test results will transfer automatically so you can see how different foods affect your chemistry and how you feel. You will also find charts that can show you where your chemistry is now, and what foods can help offset imbalances so your metabolism moves you in the right direction if you are imbalanced.

It is an amazing tool. The best part is that $20 per year will cover your membership dues and there is no extra charge to use the tools on the website. As an added benefit, if you decide that you need the help of a professional in your area, *The Coalition* can attach your account to a local health coach who can then see how your chemistry has been moving while you were working on your own.

The downloadable *Data Tracking Sheet* found at www.KickItNaturally.com is an adequate way to keep tabs on your chemistry; but if you really want to see the whole picture by using the graphs and other tools, *The Coalition* is the way to go. If you have an Internet connection and can afford $20 for the year, you'll want to take advantage of this arrangement. It has been a very helpful tool for *Kick It Naturally* readers. For the remainder of this book, it may sound like I'm assuming you are using the tools on *The Coalition* website because I feel like they can really help you see into your numbers and better understand your chemistry. I assume that you are using them because they are helpful tools that will make this process much easier. You can call me lazy if you like, but I tend to move toward methods that make my life easier. Monitoring measurements can validate you are going in the right direction. This gives you the discernment that can solidify your conviction to stay on course. It's easier to keep doing the right thing when your own measurements make the process become more objective instead of subjective.

Investing in your own health is as important as taking the time to read about it. Though improving the actual cause of a problem can take work and sometimes money, I always tell my clients that sooner or later you're going to pay for your health. You can pay now and the money you spend will go toward preventative measures and long-term improvement, or you can pay later and those funds will go toward holding you together or trying to repair something that has gone horribly wrong. We all pay, the option of *when* is up to us.

"If you ignore your health long enough it WILL go away."
                      - My Pen Pal

You can go directly to www.OurCoalition.org and click on Self-Monitoring Registration to take the tour of all the site has to offer.

Let's Get To Testing...

If you haven't acquired the necessary testing materials that I talked about at the end of chapter one, are you procrastinating, or are you just a really fast reader? Now is the time to have those tools so you can see where your chemistry is before I talk more about each imbalance. It's easy to listen to symptoms that go along with each imbalance and say, "Oh yeah, that's totally me, I must have that imbalance." But that's the wrong way to look at your individuality.

Let's say that you desperately need to go to Hallmark to pick up a card from their "I accidentally called my mother-in-law fat" section. When you get to the mall, the first thing you look for is the directory. Once you find Hallmark on the directory, what do you do next? That's right, you look for the "You Are Here" red dot. If you don't know where you are, how are you going to find where you need to go? Testing yourself is finding the red dot.

Some of you may not need to run all of these tests. Many of you will be able to run just a few procedures and the results will be so clear, it will give you an obvious path to follow. Others will need to use more tests, and some readers will need to seek the help of a professional who can look at other parameters of their chemistry. Many of these professionals have special equipment or software that can supply information about your chemistry beyond the methods I can provide in this book.

If any of these tests are too intimidating for you, we have an almost free 4-week digestion course at www.KickItNaturally.com that contains videos showing how to perform all of these tests. We created this course to be free for our book readers. Since we also have more advanced, paid courses, our new system requires all courses to have a fee for anyone who registers, so we made the course fifty cents, allowing anyone to cover the registration fee.

Simple Testing Procedures

It can be helpful to perform the simple self-tests on a regular basis, at least in the beginning. They are very simple and can easily fit into your current daily activities once you make them a habit. I like to see people run most of these tests at least twice a week for the first few weeks so they can get an idea of where their chemistry truly is. This becomes the "You Are Here" dot on the mall directory. However, because I am teaching you how to look at only a few parameters, it is a good idea to run these simple tests four or five times in the first week. This gives you more of a video image of how your body is operating, instead of a snapshot.

Simply perform these tests and mark the results on your *Data Tracking Sheet* or input them into the Progress Charts on *The Coalition*. On the tracking sheet, there are data boxes for twelve different testings. Each time you test yourself, just add the date and time to the top of one of the boxes and input your numbers. You see spaces for water intake, urine pH, saliva pH, breath rate and breath hold. We left a blank space below breath hold for those who may need to check their fasting glucose daily (most readers won't need to check fasting glucose every day if you're simply trying to improve constipation). In the space below breath hold you can input your blood pressure reading, which will include your systolic blood pressure (the top number), diastolic blood pressure (the number below the systolic), and your pulse (the bottom number on most automatic blood pressure cuffs).

The water intake space on the *Data Tracking Sheet* should be filled in according to how much water you have had up to the point of testing for that day. This information can be useful in helping you understand why your numbers are where they are. If your blood pressure is much lower than normal (optimal reading being 120/80), you may be able to see that you have consumed more water than normal on that day, which has washed away too many minerals and brought down your blood pressure. In any case, viewing your numbers in relation to your water intake can be helpful.

Depending on the issues you are trying to improve, you might check only your blood pressure, breath rate, or pHs on some days. That is acceptable and any information is helpful in my book. (Wait a minute; this is my book, so I guess that goes without saying.) Always put the date and time at the top of each box and fill in test results from that time only. It's okay to leave blanks when you don't run all of the tests. When you use the tracking tools on *The Coalition*, you will also have the option to input only a pH or blood pressure reading if that is all you test that day.

pH of Urine and Saliva

It is best if you don't test your urine pH right when you wake up. The first morning urine test, while being a valid test, takes greater discretion to sort out the results because you are unloading the previous day's "metabolic debt," those acids you accumulated through the previous day. Understanding the results of that first morning test is quite complicated and I don't cover that in this book. Testing your urine and saliva pH either just before lunch or just before dinner (ideally at least two hours since you have eaten any food) will be an easier test to discern what the numbers are showing.

Urine pH

Hold the test strip in your urine stream for a second and read the result against the color chart found on the packaging. If the chart reads in half-point increments, and your reading is between two colors, make an estimate for your reading. For example, if the color on your pH strip falls between 6 and 6.5, make a guess and say 6.3 or wherever you think it lands. Just pick a number and don't say "really green" or "very yellow," because that is too subjective. Pick a number; you are simply looking for a range. If the actual reading is off by a little bit, that's okay. You won't be using NASA equipment here and you're not going to get an exact reading. You just want to be able to see, "Is it high or is it low? How high or low is it?" So, don't drive yourself nuts and think that you have to pull out the magnifying glass and read the strip under indoor lighting that mimics the sun at high noon. Just look at the pee on the strip and mark it down.

Saliva pH

Try not to drink or have anything in your mouth for 20 minutes before testing, and ideally you want to wait approximately two hours after eating. Testing your saliva at the same time as your urine will keep everything simple. Don't use the same strip for both—it makes me sad that I feel like I need to explain that (however I do know one person who takes a pair of scissors and splits the strip long ways to get twice as many measurements out of a pack). Bring up a little saliva between your lips and run the test strip across your lips and through the saliva. Read against the chart right away. Timing is important. The CO_2 in your saliva will out-gas into the atmosphere. The reading will often rise the longer you wait to read it. Because of this, it is best to read the saliva as soon as you moisten the strip or you will have a less accurate reading. With urine, it is not as important to read against the chart right away.

Blood Pressure

To test your resting blood pressure, lie down and relax for two minutes or so. Perform the test on your left arm according to the directions for your blood pressure cuff. If you are using an automatic cuff, it will likely display three numbers, usually in this configuration: The top number is the systolic pressure (measure of blood pressure while the heart is beating). The middle number is the diastolic pressure (measure of blood pressure while the heart is relaxed). The bottom number is your pulse. If it is difficult for you to lie down for the reading, you can take this test in a seated, resting position.

On the Data Tracking Sheet you will see spaces for both resting and standing blood pressures. You will use the standing blood pressure slots only if you move up to the intermediate self-tests found in Appendix B.

Breath Rate

This can be difficult to test on yourself. When you're conscious of what you're doing, you might adjust your breathing, even subconsciously. Anytime you can, get someone else to count this for you so you can let your mind wander to other things and just breathe normally. Doing so will likely provide a more accurate reading. If you don't have that option, just try to count your breaths while breathing as normally as possible. Lie down and relax. Try to think of other things so that you breathe normally. Start your timer and count the number of times you inhale in 30 seconds. Double that number for the number of breaths per minute. Just be sure you don't count an inhale as one and an exhale as two. Count only the inhales. I like to continue for the entire minute to see if I get the same number the last 30 seconds as I did the first. If not, I may average the two. My preference is to use an egg timer, so you can set it for one minute and the timer will count down to zero, allowing you to count your inhales without having to worry about the timer since it will beep when the minute is up. This can be the easiest way to perform this test if you don't have someone to help you.

Breath Hold Time

Sit comfortably. Take three full, deep breaths in and out. Near the end of the fourth inhale, start your stopwatch or timer and hold your breath as long as you can. Don't pass out or turn blue or turn this into a contest you have to win. Guys will typically try to hold their breath longer, as if this is some type of macho sign. Not once have I noticed a girl across a room, walked up to her and said, "Hey, watch how long I can hold my breath." So, guys, just know that this is not as cool as you may think it to be. That being said, do hold your breath as long as you comfortably can. It's best not to look at the stopwatch while you're holding your breath. If you do, you may be inclined to turn it into a competition and hold your breath longer than you normally would.

Bonus Test - Blood Glucose

To get your fasting glucose, test before breakfast, before you drink anything other than water, and, if possible, before you brush your teeth. When you want to check your fasting glucose, it's best to leave the glucometer out where you will see it first thing in the morning so you won't forget.

If your results fall into the normal range of 70 - 90, you probably won't need to perform this test very often. If your results are over 100, you're going to want to monitor this regularly until the reading comes into range.

It is important that you wash your hands prior to testing so residues from lotions, etc. don't affect the test results. Most glucometers come with a lancing device and a few disposable lancets. This lancing device is used to poke the skin of your finger, allowing a small amount of blood to emerge. Insert a new disposable lancet into your lancing device. (Never re-use lancets. You may also be using an all-in-one disposable lancet where you just remove the plastic safety cover from the needle, cock the lancet and push a button to set it off while holding the tip to your finger.) Prick your finger and allow the blood to make a small bead. (It's best not to squeeze your finger, if you can avoid doing so, since that may give you a lower blood sugar reading.) Depending on your glucometer, either drip the blood on top of the test strip or place the test strip up against the drop of blood and it will sip the blood into the strip, like a straw. The glucometer will normally calculate the measurement for a few moments before it displays your blood glucose number.

Easy Peasy

That's it. Your testing is done. In chapter six I teach you what these simple test results can indicate in regard to your body and your physiology. You're about to know a whole bunch of stuff. And when you talk about it, you'll be able to use words that are fancier than "stuff."

Wha'd He Say?

In this chapter, you learned:
- If your chemistry or health situation is complicated, get help from a professional who understands this work. You will still be a participant in your own health.
- Correcting the actual underlying cause of a problem will take longer than the four hours it takes for a drug to kick in. Be patient.
- Go to www.OurCoalition.org to register as a member and gain access to tracking tools that will help you reach your goals.
- Try to take any tests at least two hours after a meal.
- Testing yourself is the key to understanding your next move. How do you know what to do next if you don't know where you are now?
- These tests are simple, but if they appear intimidating, go to www.KickItNaturally.com and register for the 4-week digestion course for only fifty cents. The videos in the course will help you realize the simplicity of these testing procedures.

CHAPTER SIX

Understanding Your Biological Individuality

Intro To Imbalances

This will be the most sciency chapter. You can tell how complicated it will be by my use of such a technical word as "sciency." Don't let the technical aspects scare you away. I promise to talk in stories and analogies as often as possible. Learning how to look at your own biological individuality can uncover which foods, supplements or lifestyle changes could be best for you... not your neighbor or your brother or even that dreamy kid in all the vampire movies... You.

Beyond digestive issues that may need attention, there are ten main imbalances that can occur in the body. To simplify this book, I cover only six of these imbalances because they are the ones that most commonly contribute to constipation. Understanding your optimal food choices is valuable enough to wade through some science. With that in mind, push through anything that is a little complicated and I promise I'll get back to the simple stuff in chapter eight. This is my favorite part but I tried my best not to blab on for hours. For those who want to dig in deeper, you can read Appendix C where I cover all ten imbalances. To learn about the pioneers who created the work that makes up the bulk of what I cover in this series, read *Those Who Paved the Way* in Appendix D. If you are a health care professional, or just want to learn more advanced topics to help yourself, or your family, go to www.HealthProCourse.com to check out our online course for health coaches.

I first want to teach you how to look at your self-test numbers that you learned how to find in chapter five. In that way, you'll know which imbalances you need to pay close attention to when I explain them in this chapter. For now, I'll give you a very brief introduction to each imbalance. Each imbalance has a polar opposite so I go over them in pairs.

Electrolyte Excess and Electrolyte Deficiency Imbalances

> These imbalances can indicate the level of electrolytes in the system. An Electrolyte Excess Imbalance would show that there are likely too many minerals in the system and a possible inability for the body to remove junk, often resulting in high blood pressure. Almost 50% of Americans fall into this category. Those dealing with hypertension and cardiovascular disease are often experiencing an Electrolyte Excess Imbalance.
>
> An Electrolyte Deficiency Imbalance would show a lack of mineral in the system, leaving the body without enough resources to function properly. This is a common imbalance for those with uncontrollable cravings. Depression, vertigo, menstrual or muscle cramps, or insomnia are often seen with an Electrolyte Deficiency Imbalance. PLEASE remember that these symptoms can also be caused by other imbalances for completely different reasons. Don't assume you have an imbalance because you have a symptom that often shows up with that imbalance (I will say this at least nine more times). When an individual is experiencing an electrolyte deficiency imbalance and chronic constipation, it's very important to look at HCL production. The body needs mineral resources to create HCL. If resources are low, the individual may not be able to make enough HCL. The stool will therefore lean too alkaline and move too slowly. An Electrolyte Deficiency Imbalance does not mean that poor HCL production is the cause of your constipation, but it is worth considering that low HCL could at least be a contributing factor in these cases.

Anabolic and Catabolic Imbalances

> These imbalances describe cellular permeability. Whether or not the body is in the breaking down (catabolic) or building up (anabolic) phase is a major focus when it comes to these two imbalances. Knowing cellular permeability can give you system-wide information instead of the tunnel vision that symptoms normally provide. This is also the state that can dictate whether the body will send more water to the bowels or the kidneys. When it comes to constipation, understanding if you are

dealing with a problem in this area may be the biggest factor that helps you see the results you're looking for.

Fat Burner and Carb Burner Imbalances

The body is designed to burn both fats and glucose, generally speaking. Some individuals get stuck burning more fats than glucose, or vice versa. If one of these imbalances shows as a result of your self-tests, you would likely be burning predominantly fat or glucose.

The point I drive home throughout this book is this: With just about any symptom (like constipation), there can be multiple causes. Some underlying causes can be more serious than others. Some may be easier to improve. Some may not apply to you at all. It's likely that I cover topics that will have you thinking, "What the heck does this have to do with my plugged up rear end? Why can't this idiot just get to the point?" Remember that this book is about improving health and not about fighting or beating one problem. The body is a complex machine, even more complex than an Etch-a-Sketch. (I'm really good at making the stairs.) Many issues and imbalances can have layers of causes that all need to be addressed. In that same manner, one little imbalance can throw five or six systems out of whack; and, if you can improve that one imbalance, all kinds of craziness can go back to normal.

I am about to cover how symptoms can be used as a piece of data, but that DOES NOT mean that the symptoms are the data. If you and I were standing in my kitchen talking about this right now, I would shake you just to make sure you were listening to me. I also really like to shake people while I try to make a funny point just to see if I can get away with it. In any case, pretend I just shook you so that the point about symptoms and jumping to conclusions sinks in.

With chapter five teaching you how to run simple tests, the next step is for me to help you understand how these numbers can be translated into imbalances. In other words, now we can look at how whacked you really are and why you're not the captain of regular bowel movements. Even though one of the goals of this book is to sway you from living your life through symptoms, you can still use symptoms to further understand where your body chemistry may be going awry. Symptoms become more meaningful when they are seen in a context of biological measurement. With that in mind, be certain you don't look at a symptom that is sometimes associated with an imbalance and assume you must have that imbalance. Use the numbers as your main reference point.

Imbalance Guide

On the next page, you see a copy of the *Basic Imbalance Guide* (referred to as *Imbalance Guide* for the rest of the book). If you didn't download a copy when you printed off your *Data Tracking Sheet*, you can do that now. Go to our website, www.KickItNaturally.com. Just click on BOOK TOOLS and BASIC IMBALANCE GUIDE. While you're on our site, you might also want to download our free "Quick Start Guide."

I also include here a sample *Imbalance Guide* that has been filled out. This will give you a visual of how specific results can help to determine whether or not you should circle an imbalance that needs correction or underline an imbalance that may need a little boost in the right direction. It truly can be an amazing help to actually download and print off these forms so you can hold them in your hand. By simply taking the time to fill out your numbers, you can see that this process is not as complicated as it looks at first glance. If you run into trouble, be sure to join the private Facebook group so you can ask questions.

www.Facebook.com/groups/kickyourfatsupport/

This page left blank intentionally so that your Sample Imbalance Guide and Sample Completed Imbalance Guide can appear side by side on the following pages.

*You can use this space to color if you like.
Maybe you'll color a pony.*

IMBALANCE GUIDE

Name: _____   Date: _____ Time: _____

Electrolyte Status

Systolic	<	92	97	102	107	112		130	135	140	145	150	>

Electrolyte Deficiency Imbalance	Balanced 112/74 - 130/87	Electrolyte Excess Imbalance

Diastolic	<	54	59	64	69	74		87	92	97	102	107	>

Circle Your Breath Rate

Less Than 10 — See Appendix C   10 11 12 13 14 15 16 17 18 19 20   More Than 20 — See Appendix C

Breath Hold Time = _____ Seconds

Catabolic/Anabolic Validators

Catabolic	Anabolic
__ Urine pH < 6.1	Urine pH > 6.3 __
__ Saliva pH > 6.9	Saliva pH < 6.6 __
__ Oliguria	Polyuria __
__ Soft/Loose Stool	Hard Stool / Constipation __
__ Wake Easily	Difficult to Rise __
__ High Debris in Urine	Low Debris in Urine __
__ Migraines	Anxiety __

pH Chart

Urine   Saliva

8.0
May Push urine pH down — Monitor to Validate   May Push Saliva pH down — Monitor to Validate

Organ Meats
Vitamin C as ascorbic acid

Sauerkraut
Yogurt
Betaine HCL
Cayenne Pepper Capsules
Lemon in Water

7.5

Energy Validators

Fat Burner	Carb Burner
__ Breath Rate < 15bpm	Breath Rate > 16bpm __
__ Breath Hold > 50sec	Breath Hold < 50sec __
__ Systolic BP > 133	Systolic BP < 112 __
__ Glucose > 100	Glucose < 70 __
__ Urine pH < 6.1	Urine pH > 6.3 __
__ Saliva pH > 6.9	Saliva pH < 6.6 __
__ Type II Diabetes	Irritable When Hungry __

7.0

6.5

6.0
5.8 - 6.3 Optimal Zone When Breath Rate is 16-20

5.5 - 6.0 Optimal Zone When Breath Rate is 10-15

Vitamin B12
Digestive Enzymes
CoQ10

Digestive Issue Validators

__ Systolic Blood Pressure < 112
__ Diastolic Blood Pressure < 74
__ Burping and/or Bloating
__ Passing Gas
__ Reflux/Heartburn
__ Light Colored Stool
__ Constipation
__ Urgent Diarrhea
__ Nausea

5.5
Butter
Coconut Oil

Cottage Cheese
Corn Meal
Lima Beans
Buckwheat
Squash

5.0
May Push urine pH up — Monitor to Validate   May Push Saliva pH up — Monitor to Validate

▨ = My Optimal Zones

Needs Improvement

| Electrolyte Deficiency | Anabolic | Carb Burner | |
| Electrolyte Excess | Catabolic | Fat Burner | Digestive Issues |

78

Sample Completed *Imbalance Guide*

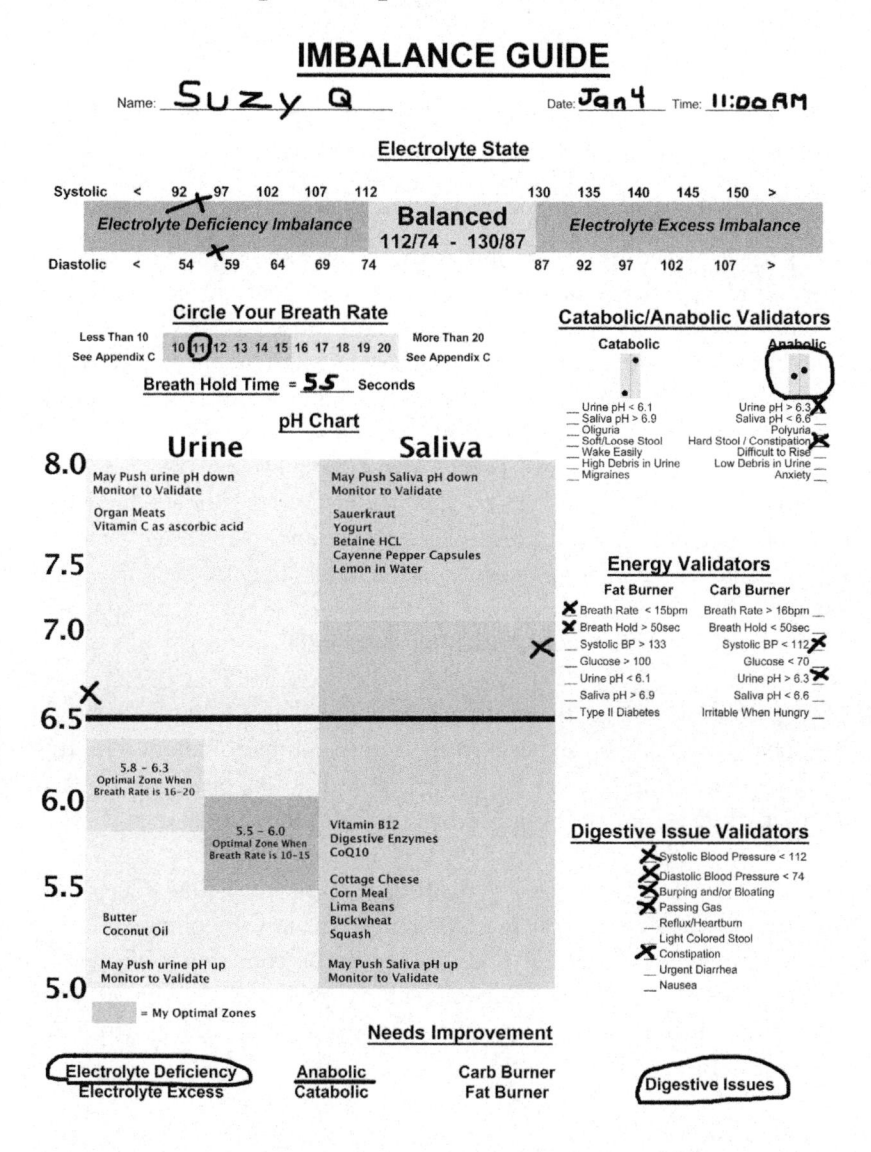

IMBALANCE GUIDE

Name: **Suzy Q**　　　　Date: **Jan 4**　Time: **11:00 AM**

Electrolyte State

| Systolic < | 92 | 97 | 102 | 107 | 112 | | 130 | 135 | 140 | 145 | 150 | > |

Electrolyte Deficiency Imbalance | **Balanced 112/74 - 130/87** | *Electrolyte Excess Imbalance*

| Diastolic < | 54 | 59 | 64 | 69 | 74 | | 87 | 92 | 97 | 102 | 107 | > |

Circle Your Breath Rate

Less Than 10 — See Appendix C　　10 **11** 12 13 14 15 16 17 18 19 20　　More Than 20 — See Appendix C

Breath Hold Time = 55 Seconds

Catabolic/Anabolic Validators

Catabolic　　　　**Anabolic** (circled)

- __ Urine pH < 6.1　　　✗ Urine pH > 6.3
- __ Saliva pH > 6.9　　　__ Saliva pH < 6.6
- __ Oliguria　　　　　　　✗ Polyuria
- __ Soft/Loose Stool　　　__ Hard Stool / Constipation
- __ Wake Easily　　　　　__ Difficult to Rise
- __ High Debris in Urine　__ Low Debris in Urine
- __ Migraines　　　　　　__ Anxiety

pH Chart

Urine | **Saliva**

8.0 — May Push urine pH down / Monitor to Validate | May Push Saliva pH down / Monitor to Validate

Organ Meats / Vitamin C as ascorbic acid | Sauerkraut / Yogurt / Betaine HCL

7.5 | Cayenne Pepper Capsules / Lemon in Water

Energy Validators

Fat Burner	Carb Burner
✗ Breath Rate < 15bpm	__ Breath Rate > 16bpm
✗ Breath Hold > 50sec	__ Breath Hold < 50sec
__ Systolic BP > 133	✗ Systolic BP < 112
__ Glucose > 100	__ Glucose < 70
__ Urine pH < 6.1	✗ Urine pH > 6.3
__ Saliva pH > 6.9	__ Saliva pH < 6.6
__ Type II Diabetes	__ Irritable When Hungry

7.0 — ✗ (mark in Saliva column)

6.5 — ✗ (mark in Urine column)

6.0 — 5.8 - 6.3 Optimal Zone When Breath Rate is 16-20

5.5 — 5.5 - 6.0 Optimal Zone When Breath Rate is 10-15 | Vitamin B12 / Digestive Enzymes / CoQ10

Butter / Coconut Oil | Cottage Cheese / Corn Meal / Lima Beans / Buckwheat / Squash

5.0 — May Push urine pH up / Monitor to Validate | May Push Saliva pH up / Monitor to Validate

Digestive Issue Validators

- ✗ Systolic Blood Pressure < 112
- ✗ Diastolic Blood Pressure < 74
- ✗ Burping and/or Bloating
- ✗ Passing Gas
- __ Reflux/Heartburn
- __ Light Colored Stool
- ✗ Constipation
- __ Urgent Diarrhea
- __ Nausea

▓ = My Optimal Zones

Needs Improvement

| (**Electrolyte Deficiency**) | Anabolic | Carb Burner | (**Digestive Issues**) |
| Electrolyte Excess | Catabolic | Fat Burner | |

You should already have numbers on your *Data Tracking Sheet* from your self-tests. If you don't, what's the holdup? Are you trying to hurt me? Simply take the numbers from your *Data Tracking Sheet* and fill in your *Imbalance Guide*. If any of these steps seem too complicated, there is a great video in our fifty cent 4-Week Digestion course at www.KickItNaturally.com. Here is the easy breakdown:

Electrolyte State

On the red and green electrolyte state bar, according to your blood pressure reading, mark an "X" on the top of the bar, and another "X" on the bottom. The top "X" coincides with your systolic (top) blood pressure reading. The bottom "X" coincides with your diastolic (bottom) blood pressure reading. (Remember that "top" and "bottom" refer to systolic and diastolic, respectively. Yet, on most automatic blood pressure cuffs the very bottom number is your pulse.)
This section indicates if your electrolyte state is balanced, electrolyte deficient or electrolyte excess. The green zone is an optimal blood pressure reading of 112/74 to 130/90. If both of your "X" marks fall in the red zone on the left, that could indicate an Electrolyte Deficiency Imbalance. If both of your "X" marks fall in the red zone on the right, this could indicate an Electrolyte Excess Imbalance. In either case, the distance from the balanced green zone counts. If your systolic blood pressure is 165, that is quite a bit higher than 130 and a person may consider this an area that could use a lot of attention.

If only the top number or the bottom number pushes into the left or right red zones, you may be experiencing only a slight imbalance in that direction. For example, if your systolic pressure is 105, but your diastolic is 78, there may be only a slight Electrolyte Deficiency Imbalance.

Special note: If your systolic reading falls within the Electrolyte Deficiency Imbalance box on the left, yet your diastolic blood pressure (bottom number) is above 89, you would not be considered electrolyte deficient. However, if your diastolic blood pressure is over 90 on a regular basis, it may be time to have your doctor or health practitioner check that out.

A Word On Medications

If your systolic blood pressure is in the green zone, yet you are currently taking blood pressure lowering medications, you're really not that balanced at all, are you? If your doctor felt like you needed to be on blood pressure meds, odds are pretty great that you are experiencing an Electrolyte Excess Imbalance.

The same thing goes for the other direction. If you show a balanced blood pressure number, yet you're currently taking antidepressants, you may be dealing with an Electrolyte Deficiency Imbalance since depression medications can often restrict a person's ability to pee out salts, thereby raising blood pressure, in most cases.

Breath Rate and Breath Hold Time

Circle the number that corresponds with your breaths per minute (remember, you are counting only inhales, not inhales and exhales). You will use this information to determine your optimal urine pH zone. If your breath rate is below 10 or above 20, that's a problem. You may not need to call 911, but you do need to read *pH Balance - Acid/Alkaline Imbalances* in Appendix C. Taking steps to improve an abnormal breath rate can bring about a great deal of relief to someone who has been suffering for a long time.

Next to Breath Hold Time, simply fill in the number of seconds you were able to comfortably hold your breath.

Catabolic/Anabolic State

On your *Imbalance Guide*, notice the heading, pH Chart. For both urine and saliva you see optimal green zones. This is where most people want their pHs to fall. There are two different green zones for urine that overlap because the optimal zone for urine pH changes according to your breath rate. In this regard, if your breath rate changes due to nutritional changes you make, be sure to shoot for the optimal green zone according to your breath rate. *The Coalition* has an amazing tool called a pH Balancing Chart that changes the green zones for you automatically. I teach you how to use that later in this chapter.

Look at the urine and saliva pH numbers that you recorded on your *Data Tracking Sheet* and place an "X" for each of those numbers onto the pH Chart. If either of your pHs fall outside of those optimal zones, you may want to give this area some attention. If your pHs fall within both green zones, you may be balanced in this area. It's okay to be balanced; that is what you're shooting for.

You also see foods or supplements listed in each quadrant of the pH chart. The top left quadrant lists foods or supplements that may enable urine pH to come down. The bottom left are items that can enable urine pH to come up. The same idea occurs on the right side for saliva. With these guides, you can see which foods or supplements may help push you closer to a balanced state.

Under Catabolic/Anabolic Validators on your *Imbalance Guide*, below each heading you see a box that represents sample pH readings that are common for each imbalance. With an Anabolic Imbalance, urine pH is commonly higher and closer to the saliva pH reading. With a Catabolic Imbalance, the urine pH is commonly lower and further away from the saliva reading. In other words, in a Catabolic Imbalance, there is more distance between the urine and saliva pH numbers.

Below these sample readings are common symptoms that can accompany each imbalance. Check off any that frequently apply to you. Again, don't assume you have an imbalance just because you experience the symptoms. Use the symptoms only as validation of what the numbers are indicating as a possible imbalance.

Special Notes

1. Under "Catabolic," oliguria means that you do not urinate frequently, or maybe you urinate frequently, but in small amounts. Under "Anabolic," polyuria means you urinate frequently, with volume.
2. High or low debris in urine is asking, if you pee in a cup, do you see a lot of debris particles dispersed in your urine?
3. On the catabolic side, check off "Migraines" only if your headaches frequently originate in the back of your head or neck. If you get frontal headaches, those are not generally migraines and you should not check this box.

Energy Production

Under Energy Validators, check off the points that are appropriate for you, whether they be numbers from your self-tests or symptoms you experience. If you were unable to run some of the numbers, like glucose, leave that space blank and simply use the data that you do have.

If one side shows a predominant number of checks, you may be experiencing that imbalance. If checks are distributed fairly evenly between both sides, then you are likely balanced in your energy production and that is a good thing. Concern yourself with one of these imbalances only if you appear to sway strongly in one direction. For example, if you have five or six items checked on one side and maybe only one or two on the other.

Digestive Issues

If you can check off any of the items listed under Digestive Issues, it would be wise to focus on improving digestion.

Conclusions

Finally, draw some type of conclusion. Any conclusions you find may change as you make adjustments to your nutrition, however, the idea is to come to a conclusion. Are you balanced in all areas? Do you need a lot of attention in the area of electrolytes but everything else looks good? Where are you? Come to a conclusion so you will know which imbalances to pay attention to while I explain them in the next chapter.

Under the Needs Improvement section, select any imbalances that you feel could use help. If you feel that the imbalance is strong (or severe) and needs a lot of work, you can circle that imbalance. If you feel that the imbalance is present, but could maybe just use a little attention, you can underline that imbalance. Keep this *Imbalance Guide* handy while you read through the rest of the book so you can remember which imbalances need attention. This will be helpful as I go over foods and supplement choices that can be used to improve specific imbalances.

Keep in mind that the tools I have provided for you to get a glimpse of your chemistry will give you just that: A glimpse. I have placed intermediate testing procedures in Appendix B and people can learn even more in-depth information about their own body by working with a professional health coach. When looking at only a few biological markers, imbalances can be disguised or misinterpreted. With this in mind, I suggest only taking major steps to facilitate an imbalance moving in the optimal direction if that imbalance appears to be strong. After all, the goal should be to become balanced, not to create another imbalance in the opposite direction.

In chapter seven I explain how these imbalances can affect your health, your life and your bowel movements.

Wha'd He Say?

In this chapter, you learned:
- Interpreting your numbers on your *Imbalance Guide* is the first step toward understanding the causes for *your* constipation.
- When deciding if you are dealing with a specific imbalance or not, the measurements are your greatest influence. Symptoms should be used only as a confirmation marker. Do not mark yourself as having an imbalance simply because you are experiencing symptoms often seen with that imbalance.
- If you appear to be experiencing a strong imbalance on your *Imbalance Guide*, go to the bottom of the page and circle that imbalance. If you appear to have a slight imbalance, you can underline that imbalance at the bottom of the *Imbalance Guide*. If you appear to be balanced in that area, don't mark that imbalance at all.
- If you understand which imbalances may be giving you trouble, you will now know which information to pay more attention to for the rest of the book.

CHAPTER SEVEN

How Imbalances Contribute To Constipation

This information will be your secret weapon. Beyond improving digestion, many readers won't have a lot of imbalances that need improving. The Anabolic Imbalance will likely be a common imbalance experienced by the readers of this book. Sugar, starches and excessive carbs can all exacerbate an Anabolic Imbalance. Many things have the ability to push people toward eating more sugars and carbs. Even one of the other imbalances below can push you to consume more sugars and carbs. Therefore, identifying and correcting additional imbalances may also help.

Electrolyte State

The electrolyte state is defined by blood pressure (though a professional health coach may have equipment that can look at other variables in this equation, like conductivity of urine and saliva).

In the world of natural health, where the terrain of the body gives so many insights into how the body is functioning, if an imbalance can exist in one direction, there must be an opposite to that imbalance. Otherwise, there would be no middle ground, no place where the body could be considered "balanced." Seems reasonable, right? By the time you finish this book, you will likely realize how ridiculous it is that the medical world puts so much attention on high blood pressure, but totally ignores an equally debilitating imbalance in the other direction. Low blood pressure may not be as dangerous as high blood pressure, in many cases. However, that doesn't mean that finding relief is less important to the person suffering from the effects of low blood pressure.

Imbalance - Electrolyte Deficiency

When blood pressure is low, this is often a reflection of low mineral content in the bloodstream. When the blood pressure decreases, it is a reflection of a decrease in your salts or the vascular system being too open (dilated). Our mineral content not only comes from actual salt, but from our food too. As I covered in chapter three, if your digestion is not working properly, you can't assimilate the minerals from the food you're eating and the mineral content in the system isn't sustained. There are a few other contributing factors that could possibly result in low blood pressure and I will get back to this soon.

Very few doctors will ever talk to you about your blood pressure being low. Since there is no drug for low blood pressure, the ramifications are not in their training. We all know that high blood pressure can cause heart attacks and strokes (blowouts). When they say your blood pressure is great even though it's too low, they're saying that you'll never have a blowout. But is it fun to run around on flat tires all day? An optimal blood pressure reading is said to be 120 over 80. So, if 140 over 90 is considered high blood pressure in the medical world, wouldn't having those numbers off by the same amount in the other direction be regarded as low blood pressure? Shouldn't a reading of 100 over 70 be considered low?

The minerals, or salts, in the system represent the conductivity, or ability for electricity to flow through the system. When the mineral content is low, there's insufficient spark or electrical current; and energy can be low. Without this energy, the brain can't function at its full potential. Some people with depression, and even other manifestations of "mental illness," are often merely cases where there is not enough mineral in the system. Low mineral levels often mean there's not enough spark to give the brain what it needs to function correctly, or there is not enough mineral to control blood pH sufficiently. Of course, blood sugar is a big player in this regard also, but I get into that in a bit.

The body also needs minerals to produce HCL. Without enough HCL, the stool can move slower (as discussed in chapter four). We seem to have the mindset that, if what we're eating is providing us with enough energy to stand up and walk to our car, we have all the resources we need. But every task that our bodies handle needs resources to complete it. Vitamins, minerals, amino acids, fats—they're all important. The mineral in the system is very important because, without it, there is no way for signals to travel from the body to the brain. It's like electricity in water. If you put an electrical current in water, you get shocked and it's really not that fun. You get shocked because that water contains minerals; and that current can travel through the minerals. But if you put a current in distilled water, with no mineral in it, the current doesn't travel. It's the same way with the human brain. If signals can't travel, the brain doesn't work optimally and we feel depressed, tired, lethargic or, in the worst cases, maybe we think that we're a fire truck. Many of the clients with depression issues who have come to me and my colleagues, have shown a low blood pressure reading (unless they are taking an antidepressant that is artificially raising their blood pressure). There are exceptions to every rule. I mean just the other day I saw a guy with a mullet that actually looked good, so there can be a first time for everything. But generally speaking, the majority of clients I see with depression symptoms have low blood pressure.

The brain needs fuel just like anything else. If your toaster isn't working, what's the first thing you check? You look to see if it's plugged in. You don't send your toaster to therapy or soak it in medication; you just look to see if it's getting the juice it needs to function properly. I'm not saying that therapy can't be beneficial for some people; I'm just saying that, when it comes to mechanical objects, we have the sense to look for a malfunction and try to figure out what is causing that object to function at a substandard level. However, when it comes to people, we don't check to see if they have the resources for their "machine" to perform optimally. We just assume they must have daddy abandonment issues, or felt inadequate as a child because their brother was always the first one to find the prize in the bottom of the cereal box. Yes, it can be very upsetting to think back on the terror of your brother having fun with all the press-on tattoos while you had none; but if your brain had the resources to function at its full potential, it would be easier to look past that and move on with your life, now that you're 36.

Don't feel like I'm downplaying depression issues just because I'm talking like a jackass. I've experienced these issues first-hand and they can be very troubling, confusing, and a huge pile of not-at-all-fun. They were especially confusing for me because I had always been a very positive person; then all of a sudden, I just wanted to ball up on the floor and cry at old episodes of *The Brady Bunch*. Once I understood how these issues can come out of nowhere, what imbalances most often create them, and how to improve those imbalances, I was right back to my old self and could once again laugh at the fact that it *was* Mom's favorite vase and she *did* always say 'don't play ball in the house.' (Non-Brady fans will have no idea what I'm talking about here and may think I'm a little drunk right now.) You can learn more about why this happens and how to improve these issues by going to www.KickItNaturally.com, and searching for our depression episode in the search box. But for now, I simply want to lay down a foundation that can help you understand how the body needs nourishment to do all the things it does. The body can't just show up to work every day and make it all magically happen. Resources are needed to keep your "machine" running properly.

It seems to be common for an Electrolyte Deficiency Imbalance to possibly contribute to an Anabolic Imbalance because a lack of minerals can create cravings. The body uses sugars to buffer the low minerals and the person can function and feel better. If an Electrolyte Deficiency Imbalance shows up in your numbers, you will certainly want to take steps to correct it so you can get those cravings under control. Once your body learns that junk food can thicken the blood to raise blood pressure AND trigger pleasure sensors in the brain that trick the body into thinking resources are on the way, willpower may become useless. Any wonder why people might continue to eat junk all the time if they were dealing with an Electrolyte Deficiency Imbalance? The good news is, this can be corrected. If you don't correct this issue, you may continue to crave sugars and carbs, which can push you more anabolic. Therefore, these cravings have the ability to exacerbate constipation with some people.

Since sugar (or glucose) is a factor when measuring blood pressure, understand what can happen if you begin to reduce your consumption of sugars, carbs or starches. As glucose levels come down, blood pressure will come down as well, unless you have implemented methods to raise your mineral levels. This is why, if you are experiencing an Electrolyte Deficiency Imbalance, it is so important to raise mineral levels if you want to reduce your carb intake.

Electrolyte Deficiency And Drinking Water

If an Electrolyte Deficiency Imbalance showed up on your *Imbalance Guide*, and you're a person who doesn't like drinking water, now you know why. If your mineral levels are low, drinking more water will just wash away the small amount of minerals you have. You have likely subconsciously become aware that when you drink a lot of water, you feel lousy. However, you now also have an understanding that restricting water intake can also exacerbate constipation.

This doesn't mean that you should immediately start drinking more water. It means that you need to qualify to drink more water. By improving your Electrolyte Deficiency Imbalance you will be able to begin taking in more water, and you will even likely start to enjoy drinking it. First, do the work to bring up your mineral levels, then, you can start to increase your water intake as well. This can be an excellent step toward creating relief for your constipation.

In chapter ten, when I cover supplements that can help, I will introduce you to special mineral drops that you can add to your water. Concentrace mineral drops can be purchased on Amazon.com and at most health food stores. Minerals are better assimilated by entering the body during the digestive process. Therefore, it is better to take any type of mineral supplements with food. However, by adding minerals to the water that you're drinking, it could reduce the amount of minerals that can be washed out of the body when water intake is increased. With some imbalances, you may need to limit your dose of this supplement. However, for those dealing with constipation, these mineral drops can be your best friend. If you feel like you need to increase your water intake, yet you're dealing with an Electrolyte Deficiency Imbalance, these drops could be a huge help. I cover how to use these mineral drops in great detail in chapter 10.

Imbalance - Electrolyte Excess

If an Electrolyte Deficiency Imbalance normally indicates a lack of electrolytes, the opposite would be a state where too many electrolytes are present. This is called an Electrolyte Excess Imbalance.

In general, high blood pressure can be an expression of insufficient, or lousy, kidney function. This means that, when excessive electrolytes become concentrated in the bodily fluids, it's usually a result of insufficient hydration (not drinking enough clean water) or impaired excretion of mineral salts through the kidneys. High blood pressure can also result from a constricted vascular system. In any case, electrolyte stress can lead to hypertension (high blood pressure) and other circulatory and cardiovascular problems. A vascular system that is constricted often points to an autonomic nervous system issue or a buildup on the arterial walls. (I talk more about the autonomic nervous system when I talk about Sympathetic and Parasympathetic Imbalances in Appendix C if you're interested.)

If kidneys are not working optimally or if a person is not drinking enough water to wash the junk out, excess filth will accumulate. We poop so the body can remove waste. If that function is not working properly on a daily basis, junk can accumulate and cause any number of problems. You learned in chapter two that excess filth can be stored in fat cells if the body is too overwhelmed to remove that junk. Therefore, improving this imbalance can result in a cleaner, lighter you. If your *Imbalance Guide* showed an Electrolyte Excess Imbalance, have you gotten up to go get a glass of water yet? Go!

Catabolic/Anabolic States

At the cellular level, the body is always in an anabolic or catabolic state, or in the process of switching back and forth between the two. During the day, our cells are intended to open up (much like a flower) so nutrients can get in and out more easily. This "more open" state is called a catabolic state. At night, our cells are intended to become more closed (again, like a flower) so nutrients cannot get in and out as easily. This "more closed" state is called an anabolic state. Cells don't actually open and close like a flower, this is just a "basic" view that allows us to talk about the different states of our cells. Both states are appropriate, and even necessary, for a body to function optimally. Due to many possible factors, some people can get stuck in one state and their body will not switch back and forth as intended.

To make the body operate correctly, we need to oscillate back and forth from the anabolic state at night, while we sleep and rebuild, and a catabolic state during the day, while we're active. Without this natural oscillation, many problems can occur.

Imbalance - Anabolic

First of all, there are many benefits that take place while a body is in an anabolic state. This is the state where the body engages in most of its repairing or rebuilding processes. You've probably heard the word anabolic in reference to steroids. Weightlifters take anabolic steroids in order to be in the tissue-building, anabolic state when they are not playing fair with muscle building. If a guy begins to add some muscle, he may think, "This is nice, but I'd really like to be so big that my neck completely disappears and I can no longer hold my arms down at my sides. I want my arms to always look like they are sticking straight out like Ralphie's little brother, Randy, from *A Christmas Story* when he was wearing his winter parka. That's what I want to look like." By using these anabolic steroids, this guy can keep his body in an anabolic, muscle-building state most of the time. It's true that he may not be thinking about the fact that these steroids are going to make everything on his body bigger except the one thing he truly wants to be bigger. If you think about it, isn't making everything else bigger just going to make that "one thing" seem smaller? C'mon guys, think it through before you make yourself look like an alien action figure.

I'm not trying to get as many Hulk-looking guys as possible to want to crush me. What I am trying to do is point out that, while an anabolic state can have its benefits, any state can cause problems when pushed to an extreme—even problems beyond becoming so huge that you look more like a video game character than a human. Although it is very appropriate for the cells to be in an anabolic state at night, some individuals will stay in a more anabolic state most of the time. These individuals are said to be experiencing an Anabolic Imbalance.

As I've been discussing throughout this book, this Anabolic Imbalance can also cause constipation by sending too much of the body's water to the kidneys and not enough to the bowels, making the stool harder and more difficult to move. An Anabolic Imbalance can also cause individuals to pee high volumes of urine frequently throughout the day. They will often have to get up in the middle of the night to tinkle. The majority of those reading this book will likely be experiencing an Anabolic Imbalance. Remember, you can still be constipated without experiencing an Anabolic Imbalance. But it is very common for an Anabolic Imbalance to at least be a contributing factor.

If you have chronic constipation, and your *Imbalance Guide* showed an Anabolic Imbalance, that's great news. Now, you make sense. You're not a mystery at all. When chronic constipation is being caused by an Anabolic Imbalance, that person will normally simply need to correct that imbalance and the constipation will often improve right along with it. In chapter nine, I start to show you foods that can help improve this imbalance. In chapter ten, I dig into more supplements that can help, for those who need additional steps, or who want to see results much faster.

In this anabolic state, an individual can also have a hard time dropping weight for a number of reasons. If a person is constipated, they aren't removing junk the way the body is intended to. We don't poop to support the toilet paper industry. We poop to remove junk.

Beyond the possible constipation issues, if people are stuck in the anabolic state most of the time, they can hold on to too much stuff at the cellular level. The catabolic state is where tissues break down and the body gets rid of junk. If a person never moves into the catabolic state, that trash removal part of the day isn't happening and this person can have a hard time dropping weight.

Imbalance - Catabolic

The catabolic state is where the body kind of "breaks down and cleans house," so to speak. In a catabolic state, the body is primed to use oxygen to create energy, so it is appropriate to be in a catabolic state during your waking hours to keep you going all day. This, along with what I just explained about the anabolic state, helps to show how both the anabolic and catabolic states are appropriate during the appropriate times. However, in the same way that I talked about people who lean too anabolic, some individuals will stay in a more catabolic state most of the time. These individuals are said to be experiencing a Catabolic Imbalance.

If someone is stuck in a catabolic state, it is as if the cells are too permeable and this individual will often burn up muscle and protein and even membrane fats. Breaking down tissues and muscle so they can be rebuilt is a beneficial aspect of the catabolic state, but when a person is in that state too often, for too long, that "cleaning house" process can turn into a body that is flat out falling apart. If you bulldoze your garage to add a new wing to your house, your house could increase its value. But if you knock down your garage just because you're addicted to knocking things down, your neighbors won't like you, just like you won't like your body if you're unable to move back into that "rebuilding" state. The more muscle we lose, the lower our metabolism, and we may burn less fat. A Catabolic Imbalance can cause bile to become too thick and sticky to flow properly, therefore inhibiting digestion and restricting the body's ability to remove junk. That's not good.

Insomnia is very common with a Catabolic Imbalance because the cells are more permeable, which is a characteristic of the daytime state. These people can't sleep because their bodies are still awake and operating at full speed. Most sleeping aids will knock you out in the head so you can sleep, but your body will still be wide awake all night. As a result, you might either wake up exhausted or you become tired again a few hours after waking. I guess it depends on your candle, and how short it has become by burning both ends at once. The point is, I'd like to teach you how to fix the cause of the problem instead of just selling you more candles. Please keep in mind that there are other causes of insomnia beyond a Catabolic Imbalance. To learn more about insomnia, go to www.KickItNaturally.com and search for our insomnia podcast episode.

Energy Production

The next two imbalances I cover are Fat Burner Imbalance and Carb Burner Imbalance. These deal with energy production and how the body uses food for fuel. Before I explain energy production, understand that I will be leaving out complicated methods the body can use to create energy. They are not important for this explanation and I would like to finish up and leave before my cleaning lady gets here. She dresses inappropriately for a cleaning lady and it freaks me out.

To create energy, simply speaking, our bodies burn either fat or glucose. Your body is designed to burn both types of fuel for different purposes. Despite that, changes can occur in our bodies, or in our lives, that will train our bodies to prefer one fuel over the other. The body may stop burning the other type of fuel almost entirely. You want to be able to burn both fats and glucose. If you have the ability to burn only one or the other, this could restrict your dietary choices and may sway you toward foods that could push another imbalance in the wrong direction.

For example, if you appear to have an Anabolic Imbalance, yet your body is burning more glucose than fat, that may cause you to consume more carbs and sugars. These choices can exacerbate an Anabolic

Imbalance and make it difficult to correct the underlying cause of constipation for many people.

Remember, I've greatly simplified the two imbalances below. My main concern is that you understand a body can prefer to burn one type of fuel over the other and this can affect the types of foods that may be optimal for that person to consume.

Imbalance - Carb Burner

Carb Burners are people who are predisposed to burn off all their glucose and do not seem to burn fat very well. Now, it's not that they won't burn fat, but they will always prefer to burn off all their glucose first. If these individuals try to add more fat to their diet, and reduce carbs (maybe to improve an Anabolic Imbalance), they can become tired, due to the lack of fuel that their body is predisposed to function on.

Imbalance - Fat Burner

If you find that you show indications of having a Fat Burner Imbalance, you most likely are burning much more fat than glucose. If you also have high cholesterol, high triglycerides and a high fasting glucose, any of these markers can be another indication that you are not processing glucose effectively.

Many individuals who are overweight and have this imbalance will ask, "How is it that I'm burning mostly fat but I'm still so fat?" This is because their bodies are turning almost every carb and sugar that they eat into fat. In order to process sugar or glucose, the body is having to take all sugar or glucose coming in and turn it into fat before it is able to be "burned" for energy.

Again, though these imbalances can create major problems, neither of these imbalances is of much concern when it comes to constipation, unless an imbalance is causing you to eat too many carbs or sugars, and/or pushing you too anabolic.

Using The Coalition

In chapter five I introduced you to *The Coalition for Health Education*, which can be found at www.OurCoalition.org. I recommend joining to all those who plan on monitoring their own chemistry. The tools provided to members on *The Coalition* website are by far the best tracking and monitoring tools of their kind available to consumers. If you plan to use the guidelines presented in this book without monitoring your own chemistry, you might be disappointed by your results. Without watching what your numbers do, how are you going to know when to adjust the things you are implementing to balance your body? How are you going to know if you're making progress and how are you going to know when it's time to slow your efforts so you don't create an imbalance in the other direction? You have to monitor. You have to be a participant in your own health. A monitoring device is not something you own and ignore like the treadmill you hang your clothes on. A monitoring device is something you actively use. The days of allowing someone to tell you, "Take these symptom-hiding pills and come back to see me in two months" are over. You wouldn't be reading this book if you found that route worked for you. The sooner you come to the realization that you're going to have to put forth some effort, the sooner you'll improve your current circumstances and reap the rewards that come with responsible ownership of your own mechanism (by mechanism, I mean YOU).

Once you have an indication of what imbalances are giving you the most trouble, you can log in to your account on *The Coalition* and begin learning more about those imbalances and different ways to improve them. You can start to input your self-test numbers into the progress charts to get a visual of how your numbers are moving and the progress you're making. There is even a graph for your "well-being" so you can monitor how the way you feel changes according to where your chemistry is. As you learn where your body seems to function optimally, you can start to understand how to keep your chemistry in the place where you feel the best. Is that like cheating or what? I just love how sneaky that is, to look inside your own body and know exactly what is needed to feel your best. Who knew we would ever be able to do that?

The Coalition also provides you with a food journal system like no other. For each day, you can input what you're eating, how you're feeling, any symptoms that have come up or improved, etc. Then, when you enter self-test results in your progress charts, those results also show up in your food journal next to the appropriate time. Now, you can look at the foods you eat and see how those foods affect your chemistry and how you feel later that day. This can really help you pinpoint the foods and choices that are working best for you. No more throwing darts blindly at the menu of life. This can give you a clear-cut visual of the optimal diet for you... and you're in charge of the menu.

The jewel of *The Coalition* is the pH Balancing Chart. This is some good stuff. As I described in chapter six, your urine pH has an optimal zone that changes according to your breath rate. If your breath rate is above sixteen, you will normally do well with a urine pH between 5.8 and 6.3 and a saliva pH between 6.5 and 7.0. If your breath rate is below 16, you will normally do well with a urine pH between 5.5 and 6.0 and a saliva pH between 6.5 and 7.0.

The pH Balancing Chart on *The Coalition* maps all that for you. Once you enter at least one urine pH entry and one saliva pH entry and one breath rate and breath hold entry, the system will create your pH balancing chart and display it within your personalized site. This chart will show you your optimal pH zones for both urine and saliva, and bring in your most recent pH entries from your progress charts so you can see if you're in your optimal zones or not. If you're out of your optimal zones, the chart lists foods and supplements that may help your body move closer to a balanced state. It's an amazing tool and worth ten times the price of admission all by itself. Since I assisted *The Coalition* in creating this particular gadget, if it helps you improve your health as much as I believe it will, I think you should show your appreciation by sending me a new pair of flip-flops. I have a really hard time picking out flip-flops, but when they come to me as a gift I always seem to enjoy them.

Improving Imbalances

Throughout the rest of the book I provide you with ways to improve all six of these imbalances. Be patient, these imbalances were not created in a week and you will not likely correct them in a week. However, for some issues that come with these imbalances, I will be able to teach you methods that could bring improvement quickly.

Wha'd He Say?

In this chapter, you learned:
- Don't forget about digestive issues. If you're a person who is dealing with chronic constipation, some type of digestive issue is very often contributing in some way.
- You MUST monitor your progress. If you don't monitor while trying to improve an imbalance, you won't know when it's time to reduce your efforts, and you may create an imbalance in the other direction. Balance is the key.

CHAPTER EIGHT

What Else Can Help?

Improving digestion and correcting any imbalances are your biggest initial steps. Those are the things that are going to bring the most number of people the greatest results. That doesn't mean that some other step in this book isn't going to be your most effective change, it just means that for most people, those initial things are key. Now let's look at what else can improve constipation and even your health in general. Some of these things are not normally enough to improve chronic constipation on their own; yet, implementing the information in this chapter can make everything else more effective. Once this information is under your belt, you can move into finding foods that can help correct your imbalances in the following chapter.

Fiber

If you've been looking for answers to constipation, you've probably already had at least thirty different sources tell you to increase your fiber. This alone almost never relieves chronic constipation. However, it can help once you handle any imbalances or digestive issues.

If you make the change to eating more real food, rather than processed junk, odds are great that you will already be increasing your fiber. This can be an important factor when it comes to regularity in the bathroom. Fiber helps the body gather up the garbage and push it out the back door.

As crucial as fiber can be for your health, that doesn't mean that all high-fiber foods are good choices. Most foods that are advertised as "high fiber" also contain a ridiculous amount of carbs. If you're dealing with an Anabolic Imbalance, you may want more fiber, but you don't want to consume so many carbs that you exacerbate that imbalance. Remember, high levels of carbs or sugars can push a person more anabolic.

All green leafy vegetables are excellent sources of good fiber. I also like my clients to use fiber supplements. It's so easy to pop a few fiber capsules when you wake up and before you go to bed; you add a big fiber boost with very little effort.

Water

Water is a pretty big deal when discussing constipation. The body is 70% water and is based on aqueous chemistry; it doesn't work too well without the aqueous. If an Electrolyte Deficiency Imbalance showed up on your *Imbalance Guide,* don't forget that you might not qualify to drink more water. Remember to first bring up your mineral levels by correcting digestion, adding unrefined salt, and/or using supplements described in chapter ten that can lift your blood pressure. At that point, you can start to increase your water intake.

Be mindful, though, that if you start to feel lousy, check your blood pressure to see if it has gone down because you may be increasing water intake faster than you are lifting your mineral content. Common symptoms that can show up when blood pressure is dipping too low include: fatigue, dizzy spells, depression, elevated emotions, anxiety, insomnia, and cravings.

For those of you with an Electrolyte Excess Imbalance, water can be your best friend. If your blood pressure is high, odds are great that you're not drinking enough pure water. Still, all water is not created equal. Since the body uses water to help remove junk, don't you think it would be a good idea to drink water that is not filled with junk in the first place? If your car is covered in dirt, does it make sense to wash it off with water filled with smashed up chocolate chip cookies? Maybe if you wanted all the kids in your neighborhood licking your car, but that's weird; and I'm pretty sure you would end up with your face on some warning fliers around town. My point is: Your car wouldn't get cleaner; you would just be replacing one layer of junk with another layer of junk. With this in mind, don't view all liquid drinks as water. If you're stirring flavored powder containing sugar or artificial sweeteners into your water, or making coffee with your water, that doesn't count as water. Water is water.

Avoid Soda

Soda has different meanings or connotations in different areas of the country. I'm talking about carbonated, flavored drinks—soda pop. I advocate seltzer water or sparkling water to many clients with slower breath rates (say, below 10 breaths per minute) and especially if they're having panic attacks. Breathing into a paper bag helps retain CO_2 in the system and allows oxygen to be released to the brain. This can ease some panic attacks. Seltzer water accomplishes the same thing without the obvious inappropriateness of breathing into a paper bag. If someone is having a panic attack, Pepsi-Cola has more acid than Coca-Cola and I advocate Pepsi for the panic attack if seltzer or sparkling water is not available at the quick stop gas station.

Beyond this handy use, the average soft drinks are just a transport system for artificial sweeteners and chemicals that your body can't process. The worst part is that they also contain phosphates that have been proven to block your body's ability to assimilate nutrients. So, basically, any food that you eat along with a diet soda is not being assimilated optimally by your body. Incredible, isn't it? That affects most of the country. This info gives you some clues why so many in this country are overweight with diabetes, heart disease or cancer. Our bodies aren't getting the nutrients they need to function properly. This can often increase cravings, causing an individual to consume more sugars and carbs, possibly exacerbating an Anabolic Imbalance. No wonder so many of us are constipated.

Quitting soda can be very hard for some people. You can actually get withdrawal symptoms because the chemicals act like a drug. But once you get past eight or nine days without any soda at all, you should find it much easier to quit drinking soda completely. Your body will start to function more ideally if it has water and recognizable foods, instead of newly invented chemicals—and your cravings can stop altogether.

Most people think that they're making the healthy choice by drinking diet soda pop. In my opinion, the only ingestible substance that you can put in your body that is worse for you than diet soda is a jelly doughnut, and that's only because it's fried. The artificial sweeteners used in diet soda are directly linked to so many brain and mental issues that it's hard to keep up. Once my clients get past the initial difficult week of giving up soda, most of them lose weight; and nearly half of their nagging symptoms simply go away.

My clients with a low mineral content in their bodies seem to love soda the most and, just like smoking, have the hardest time giving it up. Soda has syrup in it that makes it thicker so the taste sticks on the tongue longer. The carbohydrates in this syrup can also make your blood thicker and raises your blood pressure. This is one of the reasons people crave it so much and have a hard time quitting. The body can use it to thicken your blood and buffer low salts and low sugars.

I have even read that, when many companies ship the concentrated syrup that goes into soda to give it that flavor and texture people can't seem to live without, the companies actually have to post a "Transporting Hazardous Substance" sign on their trucks. And we just dilute this stuff with some carbonated water and drink it? Amazing.

Removing soda pop from your diet can better help you digest your food, use the nutrients in that food, and can help every aspect of your body. For many people, nothing in this book will improve their health more than losing the soda. When you're drinking soda, not only are you bringing in junk, you're also *not* drinking water... the thing your body really needs.

Lose The Artificial Sweeteners

Anytime you see "Sugar Free" on a package, you can almost guarantee it has some type of artificial sweetener in it. That's how it still tastes good even though they took all the sugar out. The problem is that these artificial sweeteners are just that: ARTIFICIAL. Some artificial sweeteners market themselves as a natural sweetener and say that they are "made from sugar." That is crap. They are just as bad for you as aspartame. Because it's artificial, the body can't recognize it and process it properly. Now, it just becomes one more toxin that the body has to deal with.

There are also a lot of products out now sweetened with agave and honey and such. These are still high in sugars and carbs, but they are natural and better than using an artificial sweetener or refined sugar. I don't view these products as toxic; but since they can spike insulin levels, just like sugar can, I try to avoid them. Inositol, inulin, xylitol, and lo han guo are not horrible and these products will not spike insulin levels. Xylitol comes from either corn or birch trees. I'm not much of a fan of anything that comes from corn, so I prefer to use the variety that comes from birch trees, if I use it at all. I'm not a fan of sucralose.

The only sweetener that I honestly view as healthy is stevia. It's just an herb and doesn't have any effect on insulin levels. Stevia is pro-anabolic, so I don't recommend any severe anabolics using large amounts of stevia. But once you improve an Anabolic Imbalance, and your constipation issues have improved, introducing small amounts of stevia would likely be okay.

I will be honest, however, and tell you that nobody in his right mind could possibly just start using stevia. Disgusting. But here's the trick and, trust me, I have not had one single person who actually followed through with this who didn't say, "Holy cow, you're right, I really like it!" The weird thing is that they all said, "Holy Cow." Weird, huh? Anyway, you can't just start using stevia when your body is accustomed to sugar and artificial sweeteners. The trick is to use whatever you use now, and add just a little bit of stevia. You won't even taste it at first. Then, the next time, you add a little more stevia until you have it at about half and half. Then, you just start using less of your sweetener until it's gone. By that time, your taste buds will have changed and you will have acquired a taste for stevia. Just like you acquired a taste for me. Remember how you used to want to punch me in the face at the beginning of this book, but now I'm just cute? Stevia is just like that. After you get used to it, you will like it. My advice is to get the flavored drops they sell at most health food stores so you get a little bonus flavor.

I do not have any financial interest in "Nu Naturals" Stevia, but I understand the stevia leaf has two molecules in it that give us the sensation of sweet. One of those molecules has a bitter aftertaste. This particular brand is made only from the one molecule that does not have that bitterness.

Use Unrefined Salt (Sea Salt)

For people who have low mineral content and low blood pressure, a quality sea salt can literally change their life. Sea salt is, in essence, minerals from the sea. It also contains a chloride ion that is necessary for your body to make its own HCL. Without this chloride ion, people can't make enough HCL to properly digest their food. Without enough HCL properly acidifying the stomach, the stool becomes too alkaline, moves too slowly, and we get plugged up.

Some people tell me that they don't like salt. Usually this is because they have associated decreased health with using salt so they began to avoid it. However, as your body realizes, "Hey, we can really use this stuff for a lot of functions," your taste buds will change, you will begin to really like the taste and you'll even crave it.

"Flower of the Ocean" by Celtic Sea Salt is my favorite brand, but don't feel like this is your only option. Any unrefined salt or unrefined sea salt should bring you some benefits. Redmond Real Salt is a popular unrefined salt used by many health coaches. Some feel that, since the sea is polluted, it is better to use a mined salt like Redmond Real Salt. Even if you're out at a restaurant and don't have any unrefined salt available to you, normal table salt could help you out of a rough spot if you're experiencing a lot of sugar cravings.

If you can't find Celtic Sea Salt or Redmond Real Salt, most Himalayan sea salts are also good in a pinch, in my opinion. If you think I was making an idiotic pun-like joke with the "pinch" in reference to salt, I will be furious.

Knowledge

Knowledge is power, and can help more than just about anything when trying to improve your health naturally. However, as important as it is to gain knowledge, it is also important to avoid knowledge that may not be so accurate. Clinical trials can be a very misleading source of information.

A new clinical trial reported recently that high blood pressure rates would drop 68% if they would put *Alf* back on the air. I'm pretty sure I'm the only person who has ever written that statement, but it makes my point that we will believe just about anything that was discovered by a clinical trial. It's my opinion that these clinical trials are often the origin of bad information. Once you understand how every individual is different, and no two people have the same chemistry, or are able to process foods, emotions or pollutants the exact same way, we begin to see that giving a room full of people the same supplement, drug, or forcing them all to wear a Fonzie jacket, really doesn't prove anything.

When we look at results from a clinical trial, the only consistency we know across the board is that all participants were human. These days, it can even be hard to tell gender. (I learned that the hard way in Key West but I'd rather not talk about it.) We really don't know any of the important factors about these clinical trial participants. We don't know if they are digesting their food correctly. We don't know if they even have the ability to assimilate whatever substance they are testing. It's all a crapshoot. When the numbers turn out that 59% of headache sufferers improved when they ate a peanut butter and jelly sandwich at 5:30 PM every day, suddenly the world comes to a halt at 5:30 to spread a little Jif on some bread. What about the other 41% of the participants? Even if they experienced an increase in symptom severity, the trial still says PBJs help the majority of headache sufferers. Unless we're looking at a person's individual chemistry, and then taking stock of how a substance can move that chemistry while it creates changes to those symptoms, we're just cramming a hundred people in a dark closet, throwing in a Freddy Krueger mask, and then counting the number of people who pee their pants. How is this science?

The only thing we do know about a clinical trial is that it was bought and paid for by somebody. Some company (most often a pharmaceutical manufacturer) put up the money to fund this trial (and trials are not cheap) because they were hoping to create a specific result that would help them sell a drug, procedure or substance.

The lesson here about clinical trials is this: Even a Fonzie jacket can't make everybody look cool, and don't make decisions about your health based on the results of a group of people whose chemistry was unknown before the trial and remains unknown after the trial. Without a clear, chemistry-driven baseline to start from, how can you come to any conclusions about whatever it was they were testing?

Simma Down Now

People always say stress is bad for you but they never say why. Anger, stress, frustration and all those emotions seen as danger (thereby justifying a need for energy) can cause the body to lift sugar levels and hormones in your body. All these chemicals are just more garbage your body has to deal with. It's like eating a Ding Dong. When you eat processed junk food, your body has to deal with those chemicals and sugars. The chemicals created from your stress have to be dealt with by the body too. Your body can do only so much at once. If your body has to use resources to deal with these chemicals, and your resources are already low, that could restrict your body's ability to produce HCL. Remember, the body needs resources to make HCL. Poor HCL production can lead to a stool that is too alkaline and doesn't move easily. For this reason, it can be important to eat your meals in peace, rather than from the dashboard of your car.

Under stress, your body will also take blood and energy away from the digestive processes to deal with the immediate threat (the threat being whatever is causing you stress). Your body doesn't know that you're stressed merely because you're stuck in traffic. To your body, your interpretation of stress is equal to, "We're being chased by a lion so create chemicals that will help us get away from a lion." Under stress, your body will also push more glucose into the bloodstream to be used as immediate energy. When glucose levels get high, insulin has to increase to handle that glucose; and high insulin levels can push you more anabolic and can exacerbate constipation for some people. Look at that, stress is making you more constipated. For crying out loud, calm down!

I don't know how stressed you actually are. If it's a lot, start thinking about ways that you can process these stressful situations in your life in a more calming manner. Or see if you can find a little time for yourself to relax in some way, even if it's just stopping and taking a deep breath a few times a day. The body is already under a lot of stress. Not only is it stressed to remove toxins and pollutants, or fight off invaders that have set up a college party town in your body, stress can also be induced by a lack of resources. I've talked a lot in this book about different circumstances that can result in a lack of resources within the body. Well, a lack of resources is a stress to the body. "How am I going to pay $800 worth of bills with $15?" That's the type of situation your body has to figure out when it needs a large number of resources and there aren't enough coming in due to a lack of digestion or poor diet choices.

Diet choices! There's another possible stress to the body. Do you really think your body was made to consume squirt cheese? This is not food. This is not what your body was made to run on. The things we call food these days are enough to stress out any human body. Let's say you worked on an assembly line and your job was to pick up the square pegs off the conveyor belt and place them in the boxes. One day, instead of square pegs on the conveyor belt, you started seeing balloon animals. Your supervisor is nowhere to be seen. You know that if you get behind again you're going to be fired, so you just have to do the best you can at cramming the inflated poodle balloons into boxes that were made for square pegs. This would be stressful. This is what many of our bodies go through every day. The body has to figure out this scramble of, "How do I take this substance that does not contain any redeeming nutritional value and process it with a digestive system that was made to process real food?" Help your body and eat something that comes from the earth instead of from a package in a vending machine.

Wha'd He Say?

In this chapter, you learned:
- If you have an Electrolyte Deficiency Imbalance, you may need more water, but you first need to qualify to drink more water by increasing your mineral content.
- If you have an Electrolyte Excess Imbalance, you need to drink more water. No, really... shut up and drink more water.
- Soda is not water and soda is not good.
- Unrefined salt can change your life, especially if you have an Electrolyte Deficiency Imbalance.
- Fiber is not the answer for most people's constipation issues, but it can be a helpful factor.
- Clinical trials can often be misleading due to the fact that we don't know the digestive capacity or the body chemistry of those participating in the trial.
- CALM DOWN!!!

Chapter Nine

Foods Specific To You

As soon as you adopt a new base understanding that there is no diet that is right for every person, and there is no supplement that is right for every person, then you can stop throwing your time in the garbage looking for the magic diet or the "silver bullet," or the perfect "constipation fixer." There are foods and supplements that can bring about changes in your body that will make you feel as if they have a magical effect, but they won't bring about the same results for your sister or even for your neighbor who sings at the top of her lungs while you're trying to take a nap. Since these foods and supplements don't work for everyone, they're really not magic, are they? They are just the more ideal choice for you and your chemistry.

Eat Real Food

This heading may sound like I'm speaking a foreign language to some of you. When I say real food, I mean food that grew out of the ground or fell off of a tree that grew out of the ground or came from an animal that peed on the tree while it was standing on the ground. That food doesn't include ingredients that were created in a laboratory. It's just food. Vegetables, eggs, animal proteins, fruits. These are real foods. These are the things that your body recognizes as real food. Do you really think your body recognizes squirt cheese as real food?

I know a package out of the vending machine is convenient and it's cheap. But you're going to pay for it one way or the other. You can either spend your money on real food, or you can start sending your local hospital a check every month, because sooner or later, that is where your money is going to end up. This doesn't mean that you can never eat anything processed. Our bodies are designed to remove junk safely when the body is not overwhelmed. What I am saying is this: Every meal you eat that is made of real food is giving your body nutrients it can actually use (as long as you digest it). Every meal you eat that is made from processed, chemical-ridden ingredients that you can't spell, is giving your body a problem it has to deal with. Be nice to your body now and it may let you wet your pants less when you're older.

"Your body keeps an accurate journal regardless of what you write down."
- Unknown

Diet Is Determined By Strength Of Digestion

Instead of selecting your diet from the last magazine article you read, you might want to try eating according to what your digestion can handle. Yes, the goal is to correct digestive issues so you can broaden your selection. However, while you're improving your digestion, try adjusting your food selection according to your ability to digest.

If your HCL production appears to be low, proteins may be harder to digest. If your bile is not flowing properly, fats can be difficult to emulsify and process. If you've become insulin resistant or have a strong Fat Burner Imbalance, you can have a hard time correctly processing carbohydrates and you may want to reduce the amount of starches you are eating. Understanding your current situation can help you better gauge what type of foods you should avoid and what foods you should eat.

Foods That Could Help

I really like the idea of using food choices to improve imbalances. Hippocrates said, "Let your food be your medicine and your medicine be your food." Seeing how Hippocrates is considered to be the "father of western medicine," I'm pretty sure western medicine stopped listening to Daddy at some point. It seems you would have a real hard time finding a medical doctor who would give you any advice about food at all. It's true some doctors are given a poster of a food pyramid and you can even look at it on the wall while your doctor fills out your prescriptions. I have clients with Type II Diabetes who tell me that their doctors never mentioned food to them. Even with Type II Diabetes our doctors don't seem to be teaching their patients that sugars and starches have the ability to quickly raise blood sugar levels that are already too high, as levels often are in diabetics. (By the way, I love that the Hippocratic Oath is to "do no harm." Do you really want someone working on you who's trying to "do no harm?" How about someone who's trying to do some good?)

Food (or nonfood in many cases) is what fuels our bodies. If you don't think the type of fuel you eat matters, try putting anything in the gas tank of your car other than what was intended to go there: Gas. If you really don't believe me, fill your car's gas tank with Gatorade or soda or Oreo cookies and then drive back to the bookstore so you can return this book. If you make it to the store, you're right. If not, you can read the rest of this book while you wait for AAA to pick you up. Just don't get upset if the tow truck driver wants to take a picture of you so he can show all his friends the person who crammed cookies into the gas tank. We really are smarter than this as a civilization. When we think about it, it's obvious: The type of food we eat matters. It's just very hard for us to see this concept when we have been taught so many misleading theories our whole lives. After all, most of us were taught that health decisions are beyond our understanding. At least we now have the ability to open our eyes, if only a little.

Below I list food choices that can affect specific imbalances. For each imbalance, I list foods that seem to commonly improve that imbalance and other foods that appear to most frequently push a person further into that imbalance. Keep in mind that you are still an individual and foods that commonly push an imbalance one direction for most people may have an opposite reaction with you. That is why it is so important for you to monitor what you're doing and how your chemistry is moving. Because different individuals have different digestive predispositions and capacities, the same food can have a different effect on similar imbalances from person to person.

It's a lot of fun finding specific foods that can make you feel better, but most people cannot count on food alone. In nearly every case of a severe imbalance, those people's chemistries have been moving further out of balance for years or even decades. They have likely been making less than ideal choices for a long, long time. To push that chemistry back into balance, it's reasonable to think that they would have to make the right food choices for just as long, if their goal was to become balanced. That is not a scientific formula so don't hold too much weight in what I just said. It's just a good analogy. So calm down and don't try to pull out a calendar to figure out the exact day in your life when you began to eat poorly. The point I'm trying to get across is that sometimes it will take more than food alone to straighten out a severe imbalance. But in most cases, eating foods that benefit an imbalance can reduce the required effort in other areas (like supplementation) so that you can reach your goals faster.

Supplements are a much more concentrated form of specific nutrients than what can be found in most foods. Some supplements are even made of what are called "complete foods" or "whole foods." No, not from the store, Whole Foods. These phrases just mean that these supplements are made from food instead of from a synthetic, fractionated form of that nutrient. I talk more about these supplements in chapter ten. I like to see people use supplements along with the correct food choices in order to see results faster, and then gradually reduce the amount of supplements they need until they can keep their body balanced with food choices alone. With that goal in mind, I spend this chapter digging into the foods that can be beneficial for each imbalance.

My final note about this chapter goes like this: If you have a severe imbalance that may be contributing to constipation (like an Anabolic Imbalance), and you see a food listed under an "avoid" column for that imbalance, that doesn't mean you can never eat that food again. You can eat that food tomorrow if you want—you'll just be slowing down any improvements you hope to see. For example, soft-boiled eggs normally have the ability to push a person more anabolic. If you have a severe Anabolic Imbalance, the best plan is to avoid soft-boiled eggs until you become more balanced. But maybe you have a requirement in your life that makes it impossible to avoid soft-boiled eggs. Maybe you are part of a very specific religion that prays only to chickens and you feel that cooking the egg too much will bring a thunderstorm that would wipe out your crops... or something like that. (I'm pretty sure I'm not supposed to make fun of different religions but I'm going to go ahead and take my chances making fun of the "chanting to chickens, leaving the egg yolk runny" religion.) If you are a card-carrying member of the "chicken people" and still need to eat soft-boiled eggs, you can try to increase your anti-anabolic protocol in other areas to allow you to eat a food that is going to push you the wrong direction (more anabolic). Maybe you need to really increase your food intake that will push you less anabolic. Maybe you can add another supplement to make up for it.

It is optimal to avoid the foods that will make a severe imbalance worse, but you do have options. You can get creative if you feel as though removing a food is not an option for you. You will learn that even the time of day that a food or supplement is implemented matters. This may allow you to keep some of your favorite foods in the mix by simply adjusting what time of the day you eat them.

Contradictions From Imbalance To Imbalance

You may notice that if you are dealing with more than one imbalance, "foods to implement" and "foods to avoid" may contradict each other from imbalance to imbalance. For example, foods that are recommended to help an Anabolic Imbalance may also be recommended to avoid for an Electrolyte Deficiency Imbalance. If you come across a similar circumstance, you may need to see what works best for you by watching your self-test numbers when you eat these foods.

Some of you are going to take the suggestions below and turn them into "rules" rather than suggestions based on principles. Please do not allow me to be more than a friend offering suggestions to think about.

You really only need to read about the foods below that are listed under the imbalances that showed up on your *Imbalance Guide*. You can skip the rest. I don't mind if you want to read about the foods that benefit each imbalance, just don't confuse yourself by soaking in information that does not apply to you and your chemistry. I am hoping that you've already performed your self-tests and know which imbalances you are dealing with so you can at least understand which imbalances to focus on the most. If you have not run your self-tests, is it because you hate me? Run your self-tests already.

Imbalance - Electrolyte Deficiency

Avoid

- Avoid drinking too much water or being unconscious about water intake

> This doesn't mean you don't need more water, you may. However, you need to qualify to drink more water. If you have a low amount of minerals in the system, drinking a lot of water will just wash away the small amount you do have. Work on correcting digestion and increasing your unrefined salt intake and then you can increase your water as your blood pressure comes up. You can also start using the Concentrace Trace Mineral Drops that I teach you about in chapter 10.

- Avoid drinking distilled water or tap water

> Since distilled water contains no minerals, drinking it can wash minerals out without replenishing them. Chlorine and fluoride in tap water can also reduce minerals in the body since the body needs to use its mineral reserves to help safely remove the chlorine and fluoride from the body.

- Avoid eating too many sugars and especially starchy carbohydrates

Implement

- Correctly digesting your food
- Eating food

> This means eating breakfast. Often because digestion is not functioning properly, understandably, many people skip breakfast. After all, why eat protein for breakfast when it's going to make you feel miserable for the next six hours? But if the mineral level is low because of poor digestion, as digestion is repaired, something needs to be given to the body to digest. Once the body sees that it has the ability to pull nutrients out of the food you're eating, the body is going to want more of that. The goal should be to have digestion working well enough for you to have the ability to eat protein for breakfast and feel good.

- Tomatoes and/or tomato sauce

    Tomatoes have the ability to thicken your blood, thereby raising your blood pressure. If you like tomato sauce, using it is a great way to make just about any meal beneficial for an Electrolyte Deficiency Imbalance.

- Using an unrefined salt with your food

    In my opinion, when it comes to food, unrefined salt can be the most important component to implement for an Electrolyte Deficiency Imbalance. Yes, it is true that correcting any digestive issues takes center stage for this imbalance. However, if you're not getting enough chloride into your system, your body can't begin to make its own HCL in the stomach. This is often the missing factor when a person has digestive issues.

    When I have clients with extremely low blood pressure and all the numbers are pointing to a severe Electrolyte Deficiency Imbalance, I like to see them load up the unrefined salt at every meal as much as they can. I tell them that if they are eating lunch with a friend, the goal should be to use so much salt that their friend cries out, "What the hell is wrong with you?"

    Obviously, you don't want to make your food gross. Don't add so much salt that you can't get through your meal without gagging. But if you can add salt to your meal, take a bite and it still tastes okay, you might want to add a little more. Just stop before it begins to taste like a salt lick. If you don't know what a salt lick is, Google "salt lick" or "mineral lick." You will be intrigued by what you find. People use salt licks with horses a lot. It's kind of funny to see that many horse owners don't really understand why they give it to their horses. They just hear that it's beneficial so they do it. Nature photographers use a salt lick to attract wildlife. Animals will come from far and wide to load up on needed minerals. Yet, we humans still view salt as if it's a bad thing. Oops.

    The word salary even comes from "salt." In Roman times, soldiers were paid in salt. Would you go to work every day and fight for your life if you were being paid in salt? Maybe you should. Maybe your life would be better since you would probably use some of that salt.

> I'm not positive, but I believe it was Mother Theresa who once said, "Salt 'em if ya got 'em."

Imbalance - Electrolyte Excess

Avoid

- Avoid drinking tap water that is loaded with chlorine and/or fluoride

> You may notice that I recommend avoiding some of the same things for opposite imbalances. For example, I've listed avoiding tap water under Electrolyte Deficiency as well as Electrolyte Excess. Logic might tell you that if an item is bad for one imbalance, it should be good for the opposite imbalance. However, that is not always the case. It can sometimes be beneficial to avoid a specific item from imbalance to imbalance, and for totally different reasons.
>
> For an Electrolyte Deficiency Imbalance, it was recommended to avoid tap water containing chlorine or fluoride because drinking this water can strip the body of needed minerals. With an Electrolyte Excess Imbalance, tap water should also be avoided but for different reasons. If the body's waste removal systems are not working optimally, chemicals from the tap water can build up, making the bloodstream thicker and harder to keep clean. Remember, with an Electrolyte Excess Imbalance, the blood is often too thick so it doesn't help to bring in more filth and muddy up the system. Drinking adequate water is fundamental in helping the kidneys. In this regard, intake of clean water can equate to changing the bag in the vacuum cleaners of the blood.

- Avoid eating too many sugars or starchy carbohydrates

> Sugars and carbohydrates can thicken the blood; therefore, excessive consumption is not recommended with an Electrolyte Excess Imbalance. Measuring blood sugar with a glucometer can be helpful.

- Avoid taking antacids

> Antacids restrict proper digestion. Undigested foods become a waste product that the body has to deal with.

- Avoid eating polyunsaturated oils

This can include some salad dressings, margarine, mayonnaise and foods fried or cooked with vegetable oils. (Coconut oil, real butter and unheated virgin olive oil are all okay.)

Implement

- Using an unrefined salt with your food

The initial thought for someone with an Electrolyte Excess Imbalance would be to avoid salt. It is true that if you add salt with this imbalance, you will want to monitor your blood pressure and make sure it does not go up. However, if adding unrefined salt can provide the body with the chloride needed to improve HCL production, higher HCL production can improve digestion, therefore, reducing the junk in the system that was created as a result of improper digestion. Now, the body has one less burden and can focus on removing waste. This can help the body reduce blood pressure.

- Correcting any digestive issues so you can properly break down your food
- Drinking more water
- Eating a lot of low-starch green vegetables

Imbalance – Anabolic

Avoid

- Avoid foods made with hydrogenated and polyunsaturated fatty acids: Canola, corn and soy oils
- Avoid ice cream
- Avoid butter
- Avoid cream
- Avoid cheese
- Avoid juices
- Avoid foods made with sugar
- Avoid coffee
- Avoid tea
- Avoid soda

- Avoid excessive fruit
- Avoid excessive carbohydrate intake
- Avoid vinegar
- Avoid poached or soft-boiled eggs

Implement
- Non-starchy vegetables
- Unheated virgin olive oil
- Lemon juice
- Citrus fruit
- Sardines
- Fried or omelet-style eggs in the morning (not Egg-Beaters or egg whites)

> Even in a time crunch, if you make hard-boiled eggs, you can keep them in the fridge and grab one on the run in the morning. When your digestion is working correctly, a hard-boiled or hard-cooked egg can be a powerful anti-anabolic meal and can even reduce your need for anti-anabolic supplements.

Imbalance – Catabolic

Avoid
- Avoid flax seed oil
- Avoid fish oils
- Avoid DHEA (a popular supplement)
- Avoid fried foods
- Avoid canned or processed meats and fish
- Avoid foods made with hydrogenated and polyunsaturated fatty acids: Canola, corn and soy oils
- If you eat fried or hard-boiled eggs, eat them only in the morning and limit them

Implement
- Poached or soft-boiled eggs, especially at night

- Non-starchy vegetables
- Real butter/cream/whipped cream (especially in the evening)
- Fresh cheeses such as cottage, mozzarella, and cream cheese (these are not aged cheeses)
- Coconut oil

Imbalance - Carb Burner

Avoid

- Avoid sugar and similar items like corn syrup and honey
- Avoid fruit juices and large quantities of fruit
- Avoid coffee, tea, and alcohol
- Avoid eating polyunsaturated oils
    > This can include some salad dressings, margarine, mayonnaise and foods fried or cooked with vegetable oils. (Coconut oil, real butter and unheated virgin olive oil are all okay.)
- Avoid meals consisting predominantly of sugars or starches
    > It could be beneficial for you to include at least a small serving of protein and appropriate fats in each meal.

Implement

- Eating non-starch vegetables
    > Vegetables like zucchini, squash, broccoli and asparagus may be beneficial because they can provide carbs without such a high level of carbs that the meal spikes your insulin levels.
- Eating some low glycemic carbs early in the day
    > But try to avoid meals made up predominantly of carbs.
- Keeping your glucometer on you at all times
    > Knowing when your blood sugar is low (say, below 70) will allow you to manage your blood sugar instead of being at the mercy of it.

Imbalance - Fat Burner

While you are improving this imbalance, it is important to reduce your starch and sugar intake. (Keep in mind that if you experience drops in your blood sugar and you need starches or sugars from time to time in order to continue functioning, small amounts of sugar will often bring a better result than starches will. But for most people with this imbalance, limiting intake of both starches and sugars will be beneficial.) When you reduce one type of nutrient, another type must be increased to fill in the gaps. I like to increase fat intake with this imbalance since the body appears to be burning fat well. However, it is important that bile is flowing properly so you can emulsify those fats. If you increase fat intake, and bile is not flowing well, it could result in weight gain or breakouts caused by the body trying to push fats that have not been emulsified out of the body through the skin.

Avoid

- Avoid starches, sugar and similar items like corn syrup and honey
- Avoid fruit juices and large quantities of fruit
- Avoid drinking alcohol and soda
- Avoid eating polyunsaturated oils

> This can include some salad dressings, margarine, mayonnaise and foods fried or cooked with vegetable oils. (Coconut oil, real butter and unheated virgin olive oil are all okay.)

- Avoid meals consisting predominantly of sugars or starches

> It could be beneficial for you to include at least a small serving of protein and appropriate fats in each meal.

Implement

- Consuming appropriate fats

> These can include coconut oil, real butter, unheated virgin olive oil, and those found in eggs (the whole egg) or animal proteins.

- Keep your glucometer on you for measuring when your blood sugar is high or low. This will allow you to manage blood sugar instead of being at the mercy of it.

Wha'd He Say?

In this chapter, you learned:

- The diet that is right for you should be determined by your ability to digest and process different types of nutrients.
- The lists in this chapter do not provide you with the only foods you are allowed to eat. If you are experiencing a specific imbalance, eating the foods in the "Implement" list as often as you can, may improve that imbalance. Including other foods in your diet, however, is appropriate and beneficial.
- If your favorite food is listed under "Avoid" for an imbalance you are experiencing, that does not mean you can never eat that food again. Once you take the steps to improve that imbalance, you should be able to enjoy that food again in moderation.

CHAPTER TEN

Supplements That Could Help

It seems we are always hearing something good or bad about supplements in the news or in health magazines. The truth is that the media is correct in some way or another—all the good and all the bad. Since every person is different and is experiencing different imbalances, specific supplements can either correct that person's imbalance or exacerbate it. Beyond the fact that we need to use the right supplements that will benefit our biological individuality, we also need to use supplements that the body can assimilate. Many supplements on the market today are not worth the bottle they're sold in. I'll teach you what to look for and where to get quality supplements that are right for you. Since many of you will need the aid of supplements in order to improve your digestion or imbalances that could be affecting your bowel movements, don't take this information lightly. You don't want to waste your money on supplements that are not effective for you.

Finding Effective Supplements

Many supplements that you can buy in the store are junk. What's worse is it appears that some products may even be made that way intentionally. Most vitamins, minerals and herbs have the ability to move body chemistry. The problem is that most consumers don't know anything about body chemistry and what vitamins will move that chemistry which direction. Wouldn't it make sense that if the vitamin manufacturers didn't want to deal with lawsuits all day long, they could just add binders to the supplements that make them very hard to assimilate?

Binders, lubricants and fillers are often added to supplements to hold tablets together, to improve the ability of the supplements to run through the processing machinery faster and easier, or to make the supplements cheaper to manufacture. Any number of these added ingredients can reduce your body's ability to assimilate the nutrients found in those supplements. It is said that, with most consumer-based supplements, you can assimilate only between 4%-12% of what's in them. That being the case, it's difficult for people to push their chemistry the wrong way and there's no lawsuit. Whether companies are adding these binders to save money or to avoid lawsuits really doesn't matter. Either way, you still don't get an effective product or the result you're hoping to find.

There are companies that make high-quality supplements without harmful binders in them. The trick is that most of these companies sell their products only to qualified health care practitioners. In that way, if there's a lawsuit, it falls on the practitioner and not on the company. Di-calcium phosphate is a binder I like to avoid when buying supplements because it can restrict your ability to assimilate nutrients—not only from the supplement, but also from the food you're eating.

Most people choose a supplement because they read that it is good for a specific symptom. Little do they understand that a chemical imbalance is normally causing that symptom. If the supplement they choose can help correct that imbalance, they may see good results. If it doesn't, they will see bad results. Remember, one symptom can have many different underlying causes, so it is very common that two different people with the same symptom can experience very different results using the same supplement. Have I mentioned that it's not a good idea to treat your symptoms? If you don't wake up at least once in the middle of the night hearing me say, "Don't treat your symptoms," I will have failed in my efforts to teach you to look at your underlying causes measured using chemistry instead of looking at your symptoms. Since you now have a better idea of where your body chemistry is, you have an edge that most people never get to experience. Welcome to where all the cool kids hang out.

Understand this: You're not going to be able to pop a few supplements and correct everything that's been going wrong for the past fifteen years. Supplements are not witchcraft. You're going to have to find a way to eliminate some of the things that are making these imbalances worse and add in new choices that will help you correct them. Any supplement usage is just a boost to help it happen quicker. None of the supplements I talk about in this book are intended to be used indefinitely like an over-the-counter drug often can be. These supplements are meant to correct deficiency or excess issues, and then a person should reduce what they're using until they don't need them anymore. Enzymes are the only exception, as I mentioned in chapter three. Again, when people start to work on their bodies, they may need to use a lot of supplements in the beginning to get things going in the right direction; then they will be able to reduce supplements as imbalances get corrected.

What If I Hate Taking Supplements?

No problem. You always have the option to continue being miserable (yes, I understand I'm a jackass). The truth is, many people will be able to greatly improve their situation with food choices alone, or maybe just adding a good unrefined salt. I see that happen all the time. I also see people who are so screwed up, not only do they need the help of good supplements, they often need the help of a lot of them in the beginning.

Once you get in the habit of using supplements, it can be as easy as washing your hair. Yet, it's very interesting how averse some people are to using supplements at all. I have talked with people who have been suffering for years or even decades from issues like insomnia, constipation or diarrhea. They tell me that they don't like to put anything unknown in their body. That's okay. I can understand wanting to keep bad stuff out of your body. But with chronic issues like those mentioned, your body is screaming at you that things are not going as planned and it could really use some help. Take the time to learn more about supplements that could help you so you can feel good about using them.

I've already gone over why we hear so many good and bad stories about supplements. Yet, if you know which supplements are appropriate for you, and how to find the good ones, you're miles ahead of most people. Beyond all that, don't you think it's a little silly to avoid supplements because you're not sure what they're going to do to your body, yet you feel great about keeping candy bars in your desk that contain chemicals and artificial sweeteners that you *know* are harmful? It's up to you to make your own decisions. All I can do is point out how ridiculous some of your decisions are.

Don't view taking a lot of supplements as popping a bunch of pills. Many natural supplements are concentrated forms of specific nutrients, many made directly from food itself. So, you can view these supplements as part of your food. It's a much more convenient way to get the specific nutrients your body is looking for, rather than needing to shop at fifteen different farmer's markets to find a specific type of organic beet green. Who has time for that? If you view the supplements as the bane of your existence, you're obviously not going to feel good about taking them. A hatred for taking supplements could certainly reduce the benefits that those supplements could bring. However, if you view them as a convenient way to cheat and reach your goals faster, supplements can make your life a whole lot easier.

I can't recommend specific supplements to you, so don't waste your time emailing me questions about what you should be using. There are legal ramifications that don't allow me to help in that regard. But in this book, I can show you which supplements appear to help correct certain imbalances and I can even tell you what supplements I may take if I were trying to correct my own system imbalance. After you have that information you can decide for yourself if you want to try anything. Before I get into the supplements that can help improve specific imbalances, let me review the digestive supplements that seem to be beneficial for those who need to improve their digestion. A lack of HCL is not the underlying cause for everyone's constipation, but it does seem to be at least a contributing factor for the majority of those suffering from chronic constipation.

Digestive Supplement Review

www.NaturalReference.com
Brand: Empirical Labs

Betaine HCL (See the HCL warning under *Improving Your Stomach Acid* in chapter three.)
1-5 per meal (In the middle of the meal.)

Beet Flow
2-3 per meal

Digesti-zyme
1-2 per meal

Vitamin C as Ascorbic Acid (Optional Stool Acidifying Boost)
1000mg before meals

Fiber

If all you do is supplement fiber, your results may not improve drastically. But if you're doing everything else correctly, adding a fiber supplement will give your results an excellent boost. It hardly matters whether you add a fiber powder to a shake, use fiber capsules or simply focus on more fiber in your diet. Ingesting more fiber is all that counts. (Most foods that are marketed as "High In Fiber" are also high in carbs and can push you more anabolic. Increasing fiber intake through dark leafy vegetables is the best bet when trying to increase fiber through your diet.) I find that most people can use fiber capsules with the greatest level of consistency, because it's so easy. I like Fiber-Plex from Douglas Laboratories (available on www.NaturalReference.com) or Gastro Fiber from Standard Process. However, finding what floats your boat is the best way to go.

Constipation All Stars

Later in this chapter I talk about supplement winners when it comes to improving constipation. If you've already worked up to a full dose of HCL and it still doesn't appear that your stomach is acidic enough after meals, stay tuned. I go over other steps you can take when we get to section "Major Constipation Supplement Winners and Who Should Use Them" later in this chapter. For now, let's look at some supplements that can be used to improve specific imbalances.

Improving Imbalances Through Supplementation

As I go through the imbalances, I list supplements that seem to be beneficial for each imbalance. Just be sure to understand that you are responsible for your own health and you have to decide what dosage is best for you. After you begin using a supplement, don't forget how important it is to continue to run your self-tests and monitor your numbers. Monitoring your numbers can help guide you in the dose you are using for many supplements, once you understand how a supplement can affect your body chemistry.

If you are currently working with health care professionals, you should always let them know what you are considering using just to make sure it is not contradicting anything they have you using already. Below, I'm not making any suggestions to you because I don't know you. You do remember that you only bought my book and we're not really talking, right? So, I couldn't possibly have a clue what your chemistry is or how much of each supplement you should take and when. I'm sure you see that would be a ridiculous assumption. I'm just listing supplements that I have seen some people use with success.

I also list supplements that are contraindicated for each imbalance. This is very important because you don't want to try to fix one imbalance and simultaneously worsen another imbalance that showed up on your *Imbalance Guide*. For example, you may see that Vitamin E can help an Electrolyte Excess Imbalance so you decide to use it since your Electrolyte Excess Imbalance was so strong. But Vitamin E is contraindicated for an Anabolic Imbalance, so if you also showed an Anabolic Imbalance, Vitamin E could actually exacerbate that issue. Pay attention to what you're doing; and before you use a supplement to improve one imbalance, make sure it is not listed under the "avoid" section of another imbalance that showed up on your *Imbalance Guide*. This is one of the reasons why it can be so beneficial to employ the help of professional health coaches who understand these principles. Not only have they studied these principles extensively, they also have seen these fundamentals work, first hand, in their clients' efforts. So they can help you eliminate time-wasting moves.

For those of you working with a health coach, there will be a wider variety of more effective supplements available to you. Many of the higher quality supplements that are geared toward correcting the imbalances I talk about in this book are sold only through professionals. You'll need to find a health coach in your area if you feel you need to step up your game. Due to the fact that consumers can't purchase these supplements, I don't list them here.

The biggest mistake I see consumers make when it comes to supplements is that they will buy a supplement because their friend tells them it is good for a specific symptom—they'll start to use it and they will feel better. "Yay! I found something that works," they tell themselves. They will then continue to use this supplement FOREVER! No matter what. Even if the symptom comes back or gets worse, they will continue to use that supplement because they think, "Well, this helped me before so it must be something else that is causing the problem or the problem must just be escalating and now I need to add something else too." Don't do that. I've smacked people in the head for less than that. **Watch your numbers, see the patterns, and adjust what you're doing accordingly.** I can't emphasize that enough.

Before I get to the imbalances, my final point is this: Under some imbalances I list quite a few supplements that may help that imbalance. That does not mean that you should use all of those supplements just because that imbalance showed up on your *Imbalance Guide*. Unless your imbalance appears to be very strong, you might want to start with just one or two of the supplements listed under a given imbalance and then see if your self-testing numbers improve, indicating the imbalance is improving. If you don't see improvement, it might be time to add another supplement that is listed as beneficial under that imbalance.

Just pay attention to what you're doing and start slow and easy instead of throwing fifteen new supplements into your body at once.

My only exception to this slow-and-easy rule is if you are looking at digestive issues that need attention. When there are digestive issues, and it's likely there will be for most people dealing with constipation, you need to address all aspects of digestion. Don't start by using just HCL and think you can add Beet Flow later. You need to address the lack of acid and use the Beet Flow to help bile flow correctly. You also need to make sure you are using some type of digestive enzyme to fully improve digestive issues. With this understanding, it's simple to see that the "start off slowly" approach does not apply to digestion. You still want to start off slowly with your *quantities* and build your way up; but when it comes to digestion, you really want to hit all the angles from the beginning.

Imbalance - Electrolyte Deficiency

The most important factors with an Electrolyte Deficiency Imbalance are correcting digestion and adding more unrefined salt. Try to make these your priorities and add other supplements from below as secondary tools.

Often Used With This Imbalance

- **L-Tyrosine** An amino acid - Avoid with a Catabolic Imbalance. (Avoid at night.)
- **Zinc** Keep the dose low with an Anabolic Imbalance.
- **Blackstrap Molasses** Keep the dose low with an Anabolic Imbalance. (Blackstrap molasses contains many minerals, including iron.)
- **Concentrace Trace Mineral Drops** (Described below.)

Avoid With This Imbalance

- **Vitamin E**
- **L-Arginine** An amino acid.

Imbalance - Electrolyte Excess

Use water as a supplement. If you have an Electrolyte Excess Imbalance, odds are great that you are not drinking enough water. The lack of water is also likely contributing to your constipation. If you also have a Catabolic Imbalance, and if drinking more water gives you diarrhea, first improve your Catabolic Imbalance; and then you may be able to increase your water intake without inducing a loose stool. But I doubt this is the case for anyone reading this book.

Often Used With This Imbalance

- **L-Taurine** An amino acid - Avoid with a Catabolic Imbalance. (Best taken in the morning, and near lunch.)
- **Vitamin E** Avoid with an Anabolic or Carb Burner Imbalance. (Best taken with dinner.)

Avoid With This Imbalance

- **Vitamin D3**
- **L-Glutamine** An amino acid.

Imbalance – Anabolic

Remember, with individuals dealing with chronic constipation, the Anabolic Imbalance and the Electrolyte Deficiency Imbalance will show up more often than the other imbalances I list here. That doesn't mean you have to have one or both of those imbalances if you're dealing with constipation. It will simply be common for those reading this book to be dealing with an Anabolic or Electrolyte Deficiency Imbalance, or both.

Often Used With This Imbalance

- **Vitamin B12** Can also help the body burn fat. (Best taken with breakfast and/or lunch. Avoid at night.)
- **Magnesium** Magnesium is a strong anti-anabolic mineral. That is why so many people use it successfully to improve constipation issues. [They don't understand why it works, but now you do.] (Best taken with breakfast and/or lunch. Avoid at night.)
- **Vitamin A** (Best taken with breakfast and/or lunch. Avoid at night.)
- **L-Tyrosine** An amino acid. (Avoid at night.)
- **Vitamin C in the form of Ascorbic Acid** I see a lot of constipation sufferers who are dealing with an Anabolic Imbalance do very well with ascorbic acid. Taking one to two capsules between meals (or just before breakfast and just before lunch) can help acidify the stool so it can move more easily. Ascorbic acid can also lower urine pH and push a person less anabolic. This is a cheap and effective supplement that can be great for constipation when that constipation is caused by an Anabolic Imbalance. You can find it on NaturalReference.com under "Vitamin C Capsules (Ascorbic Acid)." (Normal Vitamin C will not work the same. When trying to use Vitamin C to improve constipation, you want to use some form of straight ascorbic acid. More about ascorbic acid later in this chapter.)
- **Concentrace Trace Mineral Drops** You'll learn more about these drops under *Major Constipation Supplement Winners and Who Should Use Them* below.
- **Epsom Salt** If you are very plugged up and uncomfortable, epsom salt can sometimes bring some relief. It is simply magnesium sulfate. Magnesium and sulfates are both very pro-catabolic and can send more water to the bowels. Stirring a half to a full tsp into 16 ounces of water and drinking it in the morning can help loosen a severely plugged-up bowel. This is

not something I would do on a regular basis, but epsom salt can be effective when attempting to relieve severe constipation.

Avoid With This Imbalance

- **L-Glutamine** An amino acid.
- **L-Arginine** An amino acid.
- **Vitamin E**
- **Potassium Citrate**

Imbalance – Catabolic

Don't forget about poached or soft-boiled eggs with this imbalance. Any type of egg where the yolk is still runny can benefit a Catabolic Imbalance. Be sure to use hormone-free eggs. Real butter and coconut oil can also be considered to create supplement-like, beneficial results for some people with a Catabolic Imbalance. **Removing** the use of any omega-3, omega-6, or polyunsaturated fatty acids can be just as beneficial.

Often Used With This Imbalance

- **Vitamin E** Avoid with an Electrolyte Deficiency or Carb Burner Imbalance. (Best taken with dinner, or before bed.)
- **Potassium Citrate**
- **Collagen and/or Gelatin**
- **HMB** (Best taken with dinner.)
- **Glucosomine Sulfate** Great for joint pain when dealing with a Catabolic Imbalance. (Best taken with dinner.)
- **Apple Cider Vinegar** A tablespoon with meals can aid digestion. Even adding some apple cider vinegar to water that you drink throughout the day can be beneficial to a catabolic. Be cautious using apple cider vinegar as it can create loose stool issues if your bile is not flowing properly. It also has the ability to exacerbate constipation by pushing an individual more anabolic.

Avoid With This Imbalance

- **Fatty Acids like Fish or Flax Seed Oils**
- **L-Tyrosine** An amino acid.
- **Magnesium** (Including Magnesium Malate)

- **L-Taurine** An amino acid.
- **Vitamin B12**

Imbalance - Carb Burner

Often Used With This Imbalance

- **Vitamin B12** Avoid with a Catabolic Imbalance. Can help move fat into the mitochondria to be burned for fuel. (Best taken with breakfast and/or lunch. Avoid at night.)
- **Vitamin B5** Also great for breakouts if the person is not processing fats correctly. Limit use with an Anabolic Imbalance. (Best taken at night.)

Avoid With This Imbalance

- **Vitamin D3**
- **L-Histidine** An amino acid.
- **Vitamin E**

Imbalance - Fat Burner

Often Used With This Imbalance

- **Magnesium Malate** Avoid with a Catabolic Imbalance. (Best taken with breakfast. Avoid at night.)
- **Vitamin A** Limit with a Catabolic Imbalance.
- **L-Taurine** An amino acid - Avoid with Electrolyte Deficiency or Catabolic Imbalances.
- **Folic Acid** Limit with an Anabolic Imbalance.
- **L-Tyrosine** An amino acid - Avoid with a Catabolic Imbalance. (Avoid at night.)

Avoid With This Imbalance

- **Vitamin B5**

Major Constipation Supplement Winners and Who Should Use Them

Don't be confused by the heading. Of course I'm not saying that every person with constipation should use all of the supplements on this short list. However, if any of the supplements listed below are a good match to your specific body chemistry, it is likely that they will be the star players when it comes to improving your constipation. "Then why did you have to blab so much?", you might ask. "Why not just tell me to take these four or five things?" As you'll see below, not everyone experiencing constipation can use all of these supplements. You've picked up by now that I'm all about looking at a person's chemistry and taking steps that are appropriate for that person. You're a person. Let's look and see which of these star players is appropriate for you and your chemistry.

HCL/Beet Flow/Digesti-zyme Combo

This is the baseline for anyone dealing with constipation. In most cases, a lack of HCL will be at least a contributing factor to a stool that is moving too slowly. Even if an inability to make enough stomach acid was not the initial cause of your constipation, chronic constipation in itself has the ability to lead to a decrease in acid production and perpetuate the problem further. If waste is not properly removed from the body, this junk can accumulate and create a burden on the body. Finding other ways to deal with this toxic load can take resources—resources that could have been used to make stomach acid. In this regard, it's a good idea to at least implement HCL use to see what kind of improvements come about.

I look at it this way: Even if an individual's constipation is caused almost entirely by a severe Anabolic Imbalance, increasing stomach acid could still trigger the stool to move a little faster. Remember, stool often moves at a speed directly related to its acidity level. Slightly boosting the acidity level of the stool while you're working to improve an Anabolic Imbalance could help bring about faster improvement. I view constipation as an emergency that is creating a lot of burden on the body so I like to do what I can to help relieve that burden. If individuals with severe Anabolic Imbalance truly do not need the help of HCL supplementation, once they improve their Anabolic Imbalance, the stool will likely become too loose; and they will know it's time to reduce or stop the HCL supplementation.

Vitamin C as Ascorbic Acid

Vitamin C (in the form of ascorbic acid) can be used, on a temporary basis, for relief of constipation. Vitamin C as ascorbic acid can be found at most health food stores and is affordable, in most cases. The straight ascorbic acid capsules we use from Douglas Labs run around $15 for 100 capsules and can be found on www.NaturalReference.com. The trick is to find a Vitamin C capsule (not a tablet) this is truly ascorbic acid. Many Vitamin C supplements sold today include rose hips, Ester-C or other forms of Vitamin C that don't seem to be beneficial or acidic enough when trying to eliminate constipation issues.

Not only can ascorbic acid lower urine pH, it can also slightly acidify the stool. We hear from folks who see great results taking one 1000mg capsule when they wake up and again between breakfast and lunch; others take it just before breakfast and just before lunch. Since ascorbic acid can lower urine pH, someone with a urine pH of 5.5 or lower would not want to use ascorbic acid. But for those who do take ascorbic acid, the body will normally pee out any excess ascorbic acid that cannot be used.

We need to clarify the difference of Vitamin C as ascorbic acid compared to whole Vitamin C. Taking ascorbic acid is not the same thing as taking whole Vitamin C. Ascorbic acid is just a fraction of the whole Vitamin C molecule. When ascorbic acid enters the body, other Vitamin C cofactors are pulled from your reserves and combined with the ascorbic acid so it can be used in the wide variety of ways that Vitamin C is useful to the body. For most individuals, those cofactors will run out in about two weeks. To get more whole Vitamin C into the body, we use Bio-C from Empirical Labs; Bio-C is a complete form of Vitamin C. However, on a short-term basis, ascorbic acid can be very effective at lowering urine pH and for acidifying the stool so it will move more easily. That's what we're doing here.

Additional Ascorbic Acid Benefits and Uses

By taking ascorbic acid closer to your meal (for example, before breakfast or lunch), you may find it to be helpful in acidifying the stomach. Ascorbic acid is not very effective at acidifying and breaking down your food, so I don't want you to think you can replace HCL with ascorbic acid. Ascorbic acid may, however, improve the acidification ability of the HCL you are currently making or the HCL supplementation you are adding. For example, by adding 1000mg of ascorbic acid before you eat breakfast, you may need to use only three HCL capsules instead of five to get the same acidification. If ascorbic acid is appropriate for you, test this out and see if it allows you to reduce the HCL dose you are using.

It is common for those experiencing constipation, acid reflux, and/or bloating to be experiencing a severe bacterial overgrowth in their stomach. The waste from this bacteria is often alkaline, and can further alkalize the stomach, making that environment more hospitable for the bacteria to thrive. The alkaline environment may also reduce the effectiveness of HCL your body is producing, or HCL capsules you are supplementing with at each meal. When this occurs, issues like constipation, reflux or bloating can be magnified. Adding ascorbic acid before your meal can help improve the acidification of the stomach, in some cases.

Below, I talk about using d-limonene when suspecting a severe bacterial overgrowth in the stomach. However, d-limonene is a very aggressive and pro-catabolic supplement. Many of you may benefit from first trying the more gentle approach of using ascorbic acid before meals. In many cases, by combining the ascorbic acid with the HCL capsules you are supplementing, it will be enough to properly acidify the stomach and make the environment less hospitable for the bacteria.

Tip: If you've moved up to a full dose of HCL and still experience bloating or discomfort after a meal, a dill pickle or two may be enough to do the trick. The acetic acid (vinegar) in that form of pickle may be enough to increase the acid concentration of your stomach. Of course, the goal is to concentrate on the use of HCL because that is what your stomach ordinarily uses to acidify your food. However, if your stomach is still not acidic enough, augmenting with ascorbic acid or enlisting the help of the occasional dill pickle after a meal, may be great tricks to have up your sleeve.

Magnesium

Magnesium is one of the strongest pro-catabolic minerals. If an Anabolic Imbalance is contributing to your constipation, magnesium supplementation can be one of the most effective steps you can take. Since minerals are better absorbed while the digestive process is operating at full speed, magnesium is best taken with food (Reminder: vitamins and amino acids are okay to take away from food). It is best to take any pro-catabolic mineral with breakfast or lunch, since we are intended to be more catabolic during the day. Be alert: It is common for mainstream health professionals to recommend taking magnesium at night.

One of the common causes of insomnia is a lack of minerals. For this reason, magnesium is also a popular remedy for insomnia for some people. Most people don't understand insomnia and think that the magnesium is helping them sleep because it is a "calming mineral." The reality is that the magnesium is simply helping to lift their mineral levels. When the individual's insomnia is caused by a Catabolic Imbalance (which is very common with insomnia), the pro-catabolic mineral, magnesium, will make this person's insomnia much worse. I explain this here only to remind you that it is foolish to use a supplement to "fix a symptom" instead of looking at the person to figure out what is causing the symptom in the first place. In any case, if magnesium is indeed appropriate for you and your chemistry, taking it in the early part of the day will allow you to work with the natural circadian rhythms of the body instead of against them.

When it comes to magnesium, it's the consensus of people involved in nutrition that most everyone needs some. So the issue becomes: What sort of response are you looking to obtain with the magnesium you're thinking of using?

Since magnesium is a catabolic-inducing mineral, if a person tends to be anabolic, magnesium could be recommended; in fact, for these anabolic-tending people, I generally recommend an advanced product from Empirical labs called "Flow A," which is magnesium thiosulfate. This product is available only to those working with a qualified health coach, still I mention it here to provide a better understanding of different types of magnesium. Use of this product was pioneered by Dr. Revici. The book "The Dr. who cures Cancer" by William Kelly Eidem was written about Dr. Revici. "Flow A" is usually recommended for doses in the morning and perhaps at noon because it is catabolic-inducing; it contains two catabolic-inducing minerals—magnesium and sulfur. "Flow A" is similar to the fundamental product used by Dr. Revici for handling solid tumor cancers. Certainly this product is not recommended for nighttime dosage because it will push a person toward the catabolic—and sleep will likely be inhibited. So certainly not all magnesium can be recommended to help somebody sleep.

Yet, there are other magnesium supplements that are less aggressive. Since, therapeutically, most people can benefit from at least some magnesium, magnesium malate can be helpful. Magnesium malate is bound to malic acid. Malic acid is one of the active components that helps to soften or dissolve gallstones. So if someone has some therapeutic need for magnesium, I typically turn to magnesium malate since even the leafy greens people are eating don't contain sufficient magnesium because the nutrient density is so low in most vegetables these days. However, if you are leaning too catabolic, a strong dose of magnesium could greatly exacerbate that imbalance. There is a big difference between taking a small amount of magnesium occasionally, and using a significant dose in an effort to improve an imbalance. Always monitor your chemistry to know which is right for you.

Concentrace Trace Mineral Drops

Since the mineral makeup of these drops appears to be so pro-catabolic, using these drops consistently seems to have a strong pro-catabolic effect. Since a person also has to drink more water to consume these drops, the extra water intake can be a nice bonus in regard to loosening your stool. Since you would be adding minerals to the water you'll be drinking, even those individuals with an Electrolyte Deficiency Imbalance can often get away with drinking a little more water when they are using these drops.

Because these drops appear to be so pro-catabolic, anyone experiencing a catabolic imbalance should not use these drops, or should use very small amounts and only early in the day. For many, the goal of using these drops is to help lift mineral levels. Therefore, if you are experiencing an Electrolyte Excess Imbalance, you might not want to use these drops and add more minerals into your system until that imbalance is corrected.

If you decide to use these drops, it can be beneficial to start with a very small dose. Four or five drops in a glass of water seems to be a good starting place. If you start with the 30-40 drops recommended on the label, your water could taste funny. However, if you start with a few drops, and work up to your desired dose over the span of a day or two, you probably won't notice the difference. Though the drops are not flavored, many users report liking the taste of water after adding the drops.

If your stool starts to become too loose (I know this may be a welcomed thought, but a loose stool can cause problems just like constipation can), don't forget to reduce your dose of these drops until your stool is once again firm and solid.

...and sometimes d-limonene

If a bacterial infection in the stomach is reducing your ability to acidify the food you're eating, using d-limonene can be helpful, in some cases. (Remember, many of you will prefer to try ascorbic acid before breakfast and lunch since this option is considered to be a lot more gentle. Many of you may also choose to eat a dill pickle or two after meals that leave you feeling bloated. If the dill pickle trick or ascorbic acid is not enough, taking a more aggressive approach, like d-limonene, may prove effective). Any constipation issues that are caused by a stool that is too alkaline to move properly could benefit from taking steps to further acidify the stomach. If the stomach is too alkaline, odds are great that some type of freaky bacteria has set up camp in your stomach. Using d-limonene is a great way to wipe out at least a good layer of the bacteria. Some strains of bacteria can be very difficult to completely eradicate. Learn more about h. Pylori infections in Appendix A.

It appears that d-limonene can be effective at seeping into the mucous layer in the stomach and wiping out bacteria. However, it is very pro-catabolic and should be used with caution. Most people do well if they skip a day between doses and use it only once that day, first thing in the morning, when we are intended to be more catabolic. Though d-limonene is a natural orange peel extract, to give you an idea of its effectiveness, it is also commonly used as a solvent in paint thinners. For this reason, I don't like to see people use d-limonene for the long term. I'd rather see them use it in short cycles, like the medical world might use an antibiotic. It seems that after four or five doses, most people appear to have reduced their bacterial load enough to bring about better results.

While taking d-limonene, you may burp up an orange taste from time to time. Since d-limonene is made from orange peel extracts, that makes sense. Since d-limonene is so pro-catabolic, an individual who already appears to be leaning too catabolic may want to spread their doses out even further. Taking one capsule first thing in the morning, every three or four days, may be more appropriate in these cases.

For those who have a severe bacterial overgrowth, the die-off of bacteria in your first dose may be strong enough to cause some nausea or a feeling of stomach distress. If that is the case for you, you might want to wait an extra day before taking your second dose. Reports from those who do feel any discomfort often say that the discomfort was greatly reduced in their second dose, and gone by their third.

Finding A Qualified Health Coach In Your Area

If you would like to find a qualified health coach who can help you with some of these supplement choices, go to www.OurCoalition.org and fill out the "Find a Health Coach" form. The Coalition will locate a health coach in your area who will contact you directly. If there are no professionals in your area, the Coalition can help you find a coach who works with clients through email. These "distance coaches" can help you better understand the simple tests you run on your own chemistry.

Wha'd He Say?

In this chapter, you learned:

- Supplements are beneficial only if you use quality products that can be assimilated by the body. Supplements improve one's health only if the supplement is appropriate for that person and his or her individual chemistry.
- Don't forget to handle digestive needs when choosing supplements.
- Once you begin using supplements, be sure to monitor your self-test numbers. When your chemistry becomes more balanced, adjust the supplement protocol you are using.
- If you need supplements more intensely geared to specific imbalances, find a professional health coach in your area who has access to high-quality supplements designed to improve the imbalances discussed here.

CHAPTER ELEVEN

Case Studies & FAQs

Before I dive into this chapter, let's pause and reflect on a few things:

1. Don't treat your symptoms and don't use symptoms to label yourself with an imbalance.
2. Get help. This work can get very complicated. If you run into trouble, find a health coach in your area who can help you.
3. I just want to point out that I've completed more than ten chapters of this book without once making fun of Paris Hilton or Snookie. Sometimes, I amaze even myself.

When we share case studies in webinars or on podcast episodes, I often hear back from individuals about how eye-opening it was to hear details regarding others experiences. For that reason, I want to share a few case studies here, as well as a variety of frequently asked questions. What I don't want you to do is read a case study or the answer to a common question below, and apply that to your life simply because it worked for someone else. If you were to do that, I would make you go back to chapter one and start the book over. Remember, we are all different and it's crucial to look at our own chemistry and our own circumstances before we implement any health strategy. The benefit here is to look at real life experiences and see the principles from this book in action. I want you to see how other people looked at their numbers and their circumstances and used that information to come up with a plan that was specific to them.

Equally important, I want you to take note of how the individuals in these case studies continued to monitor their numbers and make adjustments to their protocols accordingly. For example, I've discussed in this book how something as simple as Vitamin C in the form of ascorbic acid can be a very helpful piece to include in the constipation puzzle for some individuals. When supplementation with ascorbic acid successfully helps a constipated individual have a daily bowel movement, the improvements to that person's health and wellbeing can be astounding. However, if that same individual continued to take a large dose of ascorbic acid indefinitely, without occasionally monitoring their self-tests , the results in a negative direction could be just as extreme. You don't want to be the guy whose appropriate use of ascorbic acid becomes so much of a good thing that he pushes his urine pH below 5.0 or creates a chronic diarrhea issue. Chronic diarrhea can be just as problematic, if not more problematic, than chronic constipation. By monitoring your numbers (particularly urine pH in this case), and continuing to be a stoolgazer, you can make adjustments to your protocols just like the people in the case studies below.

This section will also reinforce the fact that just because something worked well for one person, doesn't mean it's right for everyone. I once met this guy, Frank, who used his blood pressure monitor to discover that by greatly increasing his water intake he could bring his high blood pressure into a good range. Through his excitement he then insisted that everyone in his family drink the same amount of water that he found to be so helpful to him. After all, it was good for him, it should be good for everyone else. Of course his daughter, who had extremely low blood pressure and hated drinking water for very good reason, didn't do well under her father's water regime. To make matters worse, Frank's daughter didn't even have the option of accessing a salt shaker because the medical advice was to keep salt out of the house. Think how much better things would have been if Frank had taught his family that they needed to figure out what would benefit each one's biological individuality.

Case Study: Stacy Peters (Her name was actually Karen Brown, but I changed it for this book so nobody would know who I was really talking about.)

Stacy was constipated to the point where, if she was pooping once a week, she reasoned things were going well. She was also bloated and experiencing occasional acid reflux. Once she understood that all three of these issues can be strong indications of a lack of stomach acid, she started using HCL with each meal. She started Beet Flow at the same time to ensure her bile would flow properly and be able to neutralize the acidic food product that would be moving from her stomach into her duodenum.

Once Stacy reached a full dose of five HCL capsules per meal, her bloating and acid reflux disappeared completely. This was great news, but Stacy's constipation had only slightly improved. She was still pooping only once, maybe twice a week at best. She was excited to improve symptoms she had dealt with for so long, but found herself falling right back into her own thought patterns of, "This must be a genetic thing. Maybe I'm just not built to have a bowel movement every day." Stacy enlisted the help of a health coach who asked to see her most recent self-test numbers. Her numbers were as follows:

Saliva pH: 6.5
Urine pH: 6.4
Blood Pressure: 97/69
Pulse: 80
Breath Rate: 17
Breath Hold: 29

With urine pH so high and so close to her saliva pH, this could be considered an anabolic indication. Her high pulse could also suggest an Anabolic Imbalance and she was waking up two or three times a night to pee. All of these factors, along with her severe constipation, led her coach to the conclusion that taking steps to improve an Anabolic Imbalance may help Stacy with her constipation issues.

As Stacy and her coach looked over Stacy's food journals, they noticed that she was eating well for breakfast and lunch (typically meals consisting of a protein and low-starch vegetables or salad), but by the time 3 pm rolled around, Stacy was giving into major cravings. Stacy would end up splurging on cookies, chips or cupcakes as a snack, and was then eating some type of starchy dinner, like pasta, bread or rice.

With a blood pressure reading as low as Stacy's (97/69), it is common for severe cravings to be a problem, especially when lowering carb intake. Because carbs and sugars can push an individual more anabolic, Stacy's uncontrollable cravings appeared to be exacerbating her severe constipation. Below I list the steps Stacy and her coach implemented and why they appeared to help in her scenario. Remember, just because these steps helped Stacy doesn't mean they will work for you. However, if you understand why one of the following steps helped to improve a specific imbalance or issue, you can use that information if your self-test measurements indicate you are likely dealing with similar circumstances.

1. Stacy continued supplementing with HCL and Beet Flow. Since the HCL appeared to be improving her bloating and acid reflux, it seemed apparent that she was benefitting from further acidifying the food in her stomach. Because her constipation improved slightly after starting the HCL, her coach suggested that continuing to acidify her stool would likely help.
2. Since Vitamin C (as ascorbic acid) has the ability to further acidify the stool, even between meals, Stacy added 1000mg before breakfast, and another 1000mg before lunch. Ascorbic acid seems to help acidify the stomach and to lower urine pH.
3. To reduce her afternoon and evening cravings, Stacy started including a snack of berries between breakfast and lunch. She also had half of a sweet potato with her lunch each day. Since Stacy's mineral levels still appeared to be low (indicated by her low blood pressure), she was trying to include more medium-carb foods earlier in the day. Medium-carb foods (like sweet potatoes, butternut squash and berries), were used to provide Stacy with carbs that could buffer her low mineral levels and help her function throughout the day. Because her body was getting more of what it needed, her late afternoon cravings simply vanished. By reducing her high carb and sugar splurges, her pHs started moving into better ranges (her urine pH went down (perhaps aided by the ascorbic acid she was taking), and her saliva pH slightly elevated), indicating she could be moving out of her Anabolic Imbalance.
4. Concentrace Trace Mineral Drops were also added to each glass of water Stacy was drinking throughout the day. These drops contain a lot of magnesium, and magnesium can be used to help move a person less anabolic. The wide variety of other minerals contained in the drops could also help to lift Stacy's mineral levels and reduce her cravings.

Within about a week, Stacy was having a bowel movement every other day. After two weeks, Stacy was pooping every day. At this point, you will notice a few changes in Stacy's self-testing numbers:

Saliva pH: 6.7 (Previously 6.5)
Urine pH: 5.8 (Previously 6.4)
Blood Pressure: 105/72 (Previously 97/69)
Pulse: 74 (Previously 80)
Breath Rate: 17 (Previously 17)

Breath Hold: 37 (Previously 29)

Because Stacy was now having a daily bowel movement, and her urine pH had dropped into a more balanced range, she reduced her ascorbic acid dose down from two 1000mg capsules per day to only one. She was able to continue her daily bowel movements with this lower dose. You'll also notice that Stacy's blood pressure came up a little bit. This rise was enough to help control her cravings, but is a reading that is still considered to be in the Electrolyte Deficient range (her systolic number was still below 112). For this reason, Stacy continued using her digestive supplements, adding the concentrated mineral drops to her water, and adding sea salt to her meals. It's very common for urine pH to show major changes faster than might be seen with blood pressure.

Remember, this is simply one person's experience. You may see improvement faster, or you may still be sitting on the toilet cursing my name a month later. I'm sure you can see by now the wide assortment of variations that could dictate the speed at which any individual could see results. Continue to monitor your numbers so you can adjust and correct along the way. If you're not working with a health coach, be sure to post your numbers in the progress charts of the Coalition website. In that way, if you decide to get help later, the history you have posted will help guide your coach toward steps that could be appropriate for you. The choices made by Stacy were the result of her conversations with her coach and his assessment of her numbers. Since no two people have identical biological chemistry, it is important to track your own numbers after a clinical decision is applied. Tracking the trends of her numbers allows Stacy to evaluate if the choices made for her are appropriate and bringing the desired results. The numbers from her self-tests also allow her and her practitioner to adjust the dosage of her supplements, which can be as important as selecting which supplements to use.

Case Study: George Clooney (Keep in mind this is not the dreamy, Academy Award winning actor, George Clooney. This is a totally different George Clooney.)

George had taken our almost-free, 4-week digestion course and was following the steps to improve his chronic constipation. Before he started, he was having a hard and difficult-to- pass bowel movement every four to five days. He posted in our free Facebook support group that he had been using the full dose of five HCL per meal for three weeks. He noted that he had not seen any improvement with his constipation, and listed his self-test numbers in hopes that someone could help him figure out why. George's numbers were as follows:

Saliva pH: 6.8
Urine pH: 6.4
Blood Pressure: 148/88
Pulse: 83
Breath Rate: 12
Breath Hold: 50

When asked if he was using any other supplements, George reported that he was taking vitamin D, since his blood tests indicated that his vitamin D levels were low. Remember that vitamin D is necessary to pull calcium from our intestinal tract into the bloodstream. However, at the high doses that are often suggested by mainstream health professionals, vitamin D can also pull calcium out of the tissues, and all kinds of other places, and hold that calcium in the bloodstream. This can thicken the blood (note that George's systolic blood pressure is higher than what most would consider to be a balanced blood pressure reading). Holding calcium in the blood can also raise urine pH as the body attempts to remove some of that excess calcium through the urine. [Notice his urine pH of 6.4 and saliva pH of 6.8. This could be considered a possible marker for an Anabolic Imbalance. However, with the understanding that his urine pH may have been higher simply because he was taking too much vitamin D, maybe he wasn't too anabolic at all.]

I talk a lot in this book about how an Anabolic Imbalance can send too much of the body's water to the kidneys, and not enough to the bowels. However, whether or not an individual is even drinking enough water has to be considered as well. When asked how much water he was drinking in a day, George suggested that he usually has a cup of coffee in the morning and another small bottle of water throughout the day. With chronic constipation, it is very common for the individual to be drinking less than enough water. Remember that it's important to look at blood pressure before dramatically increasing water intake. Since George's systolic blood pressure number is higher than what might be considered to be in a balanced range, it would appear that George could tolerate drinking more water without risking a scenario where he would be washing too much mineral out of his body.

Another member of the support group explained that if reducing his Vitamin D intake doesn't bring his urine pH into a better range, he might want to try adding 1000mg of ascorbic acid before breakfast and lunch. This would likely help reduce his urine pH and further acidify the stool.

After gathering input from a few support group members, George decided upon the following steps:

1. Yes, correcting an Anabolic Imbalance can be very helpful when it comes to helping the body send more water to the bowels and loosen up a hard stool. However, it's even more important to drink enough water in the first place. Once George understood that coffee is not the same thing as water, and that one small bottle of water per day was not enough, he was able to find places in his day to increase his water intake. One member suggested drinking a large glass of water right when he wakes up each day. In that way, instead of being utilized to help with digestion and other processes, his initial water intake could go toward helping the body wash out more junk, and possibly contribute to lowering his elevated blood pressure reading. George took that step each morning, and also implemented drinking five or six additional glasses of water each day.
2. George reduced his vitamin D intake, in an attempt to allow his blood pressure and urine pH to both come into better ranges.
3. To help acidify his stool and bring down his urine pH (since reducing his Vitamin D intake brought down his urine pH only a little bit), George used 1000mg of Vitamin C as ascorbic acid before breakfast and lunch.

George continued taking Beet Flow and HCL as he implemented these changes. He also added Digesti-zyme to further improve his digestion. He added the Digesti-zyme because he wanted to supply his body with cofactors that can be used to make more HCL naturally. By improving their ability to make more of their own HCL, many individuals can decrease their need to supplement with HCL at a faster pace.

About a week into his changes, George started having a bowel movement every two or three days, instead of every four or five. The week after that he was having a bowel movement every day. His self-test numbers indicated continued improvement. Since he was using the ascorbic acid before meals, he was able to reduce his HCL dose to 3 per meal and continue having a normal bowel movement every day. Here are George's new numbers after following this protocol for three weeks:

Saliva pH: 6.8 (Previously 6.8)
Urine pH: 5.7 (Previously 6.4)
Blood Pressure: 128/81 (Previously 148/88)
Pulse: 76 (Previously 83)
Breath Rate: 13 (Previously 12)
Breath Hold: 48 (Previously 50)

Seeing his systolic blood pressure come down to a more balanced reading, George felt that much of his success came from simply drinking enough water. His now lower urine pH of 5.7 helped him come to the assumption that he may have also reduced a slight Anabolic Imbalance and helped the body send more of that water to the colon so the stool could move with more ease.

George continued to drink more water throughout the day, but found that he was able to reduce the large amount he was drinking first thing in the morning and still keep his blood pressure down and his stool moving properly. George was also able to reduce his ascorbic acid use and simply increased it again any time he saw his urine pH go over 6.1.

By continuing to monitor his self-test numbers on his Coalition progress charts and to pay attention to his stool, he will be able to adjust what he's doing in a way that could make his constipation a thing of the past. Good job, George. Even if you're not as dreamy as Danny Ocean.

Note: The increase in water intake was appropriate for George because his elevated blood pressure reading was a strong indication for a greater need for water. However, if his blood pressure had been very low, he would have needed to take steps to lift his mineral levels before he qualified to increase his water intake so drastically.

Case Study: Jan

Jan was flipping back and forth between constipation and diarrhea. She found that her normal pattern was to experience constipation for four or five days before she switched to having diarrhea a few times per day, often for two or three days at a time. Jan hated both of these options and just wished she could have a normal, formed bowel movement, once or twice a day, like all the cool kids.

Jan heard us talking about this constipation/diarrhea combo extravaganza on one of our *Kick It Naturally* podcast episodes. In this episode we described what seems to be two of the most common causes for a person to experience both constipation and diarrhea. The underlying causes we described seemed to match Jan's circumstances and her self-test results.

In this episode, Jan learned that one possible cause can be a lack of resources restricting your ability to move back and forth between the anabolic and catabolic states. To move back and forth between the anabolic state at night and the catabolic state during the day takes adequate nutritional resources. If an individual has low resources, the body can get stuck in one state for days at a time. If you're stuck in a catabolic state, and the body is sending too much water to the bowels, diarrhea can be the result. If you're stuck in an anabolic state, and the body is sending too much of your water to the kidneys, constipation can show up.

If a low blood pressure measurement indicates a lack of resources, taking steps to lift nutritional resources can often help the body move back and forth between these two states each day. This natural oscillation can direct an appropriate amount of water to the bowels, creating a normal bowel movement.

Another possibility is undigested food rotting and fermenting in your intestinal tract. Depending on where that food is in its rotting and fermenting process, it could move slower through the system, or the toxicity could result in the body's urgency to push it out of the system quickly. Conversely, for some individuals, excessive toxins have the ability to accumulate and slow down the whole system. Working on both ends of digestion (bile flow and stomach acid levels) can often bring about improvement to the back and forth issue between constipation and diarrhea. From the previously discussed viewpoint, improving digestion also allows more nutritional resources to be absorbed from what we eat, facilitating a proper anabolic/catabolic cycle. For this reason, improving your ability to properly digest food could improve this constipation/diarrhea combo in more than one way.

Since it is very common for episodes of diarrhea to be caused by a lack of bile flow and an inability to neutralize acids leaving the stomach, Jan decided to focus on improving bile flow first. After all, if some are experiencing diarrhea, and they increase levels of stomach acid, without first improving bile flow, that could exacerbate their diarrhea. Jan's numbers also indicated that she might benefit from thinning bile so it could flow better. Her self-test numbers were as follows:

Saliva pH: 6.2
Urine pH: 6.1
Blood Pressure: 100/70
Pulse: 80
Breath Rate: 14
Breath Hold: 47

Note: Jan also used an 11-parameter urine test strip that showed bilirubin and urobilinogen. Both of these markers are strong indications that bile may not be flowing well.

Both Jan's 11-parameter test strip results, and her low saliva pH (below 6.5), were strong indications that thinning bile to help it flow better was an appropriate step. Jan was already using 3 Beet Flow per meal, so she did a Beet Flow flush on a Monday, and a Xenoplex coffee suppository on Tuesday. The order of these two steps doesn't seem to be as important as doing them one day after the other. As an alternative to the coffee suppository, performing a coffee enema would likely be just as effective. Not everyone needs to perform a Beet Flow flush/coffee suppository combo to get bile moving, but if your bile has been backed up for some time, taking these two steps together seems to be the most effective route.

Jan watched her saliva pH the day after she completed the second step (the coffee suppository). Her saliva pH rose to 6.4 on Wednesday and 6.5 by Friday. This is a great indication that her bile is starting to flow better. Because Jan showed signs of improved bile flow, she felt it was time to work on the other side of digestion: her stomach acid.

As Jan started supplementing with HCL capsules with each meal, she could feel that something was changing with her digestion. She didn't feel as lousy after most meals and the diarrhea stopped. She was having formed bowel movements, but still tending toward constipation and having a bowel movement only every two or three days. Her self-test numbers were slowly improving. Jan then started adding 1000mg of ascorbic acid before breakfast and lunch. In about two weeks, Jan was having a formed bowel movement every day, just like all the cool kids. Here are Jan's numbers three weeks after she started this protocol:

Saliva pH: 6.5 (Previously 6.2)
Urine pH: 5.9 (Previously 6.1)
Blood Pressure: 109/72 (Previously 100/70)
Pulse: 73 (Previously 80)
Breath Rate: 16 (Previously 14)
Breath Hold: 45 (Previously 47)
Note: Jan's 11-parameter urine test strip no longer showed bilirubin and urobilinogen.

Even though Jan's urine pH came down only two tenths of a point, her saliva ph came up three tenths (which can be a big jump for saliva pH). The new, broader separation between those pH numbers was a good sign that she had improved a possible Anabolic Imbalance. The raised saliva pH along with the lack of bilirubin and urobilinogen were also strong indications that bile was flowing better. Jan continued to use Beet Flow with each meal since she was still using HCL, but no longer needed to do any coffee suppositories or Beet Flow flushes. Jan continued to use the ascorbic acid before breakfast and lunch, as she found that her urine pH would go right back up when she reduced her dose. However, while using the ascorbic acid before meals, she was able to reduce her HCL dose to two capsules per meal.

If Jan's diarrhea had continued, she could have tried a Clean Sweep for thirty days, as outlined in chapter nine of my book, *Kick Your Fat in the Nuts*. I've posted this entire chapter on my site for free. Simply go to KickItNaturally.com and search for "Clean Sweep" in the search box to learn more.

FAQs

Odds are great that at least one of these questions will pop up for you while you're working to improve your constipation. I highly recommend not only reading through these, but also coming back to this page and reviewing these FAQs if you end up not seeing the results you'd like to see.

I've never had acid reflux or heartburn before. Why am I having it now that I've started taking HCL?

This is actually very common and may lead you to believe that supplementing with HCL must cause reflux. Since we're taught to turn off stomach acid when we have heartburn, it makes sense to us that adding more acid could cause heartburn if we've never experienced any reflux issues. The truth is, if you're experiencing any of the symptoms that would lead you to believe that you need to improve your HCL levels, odds are great that you've been having reflux for quite some time. The reflux may have been there, however, since stomach acid was so low (or even non-existent), there was no acid coming up with the reflux. No acid to burn you means no heartburn symptoms. The problem is, our stomachs also contain digestive enzymes that are made to break down protein. Well, guess what your esophagus is made of: protein. In this regard, even if you never feel heartburn, or even if you're taking a medication that has turned off your stomach acid, you could still be damaging your esophagus if enzymes are refluxing back up your esophagus and breaking down those tissues. Certainly, enzymes would not damage the esophagus as quickly as stomach acid could. But over time, those enzymes could be very problematic. Especially if we feel like we've handled the problem by taking our PPI medication religiously.

If you often experience burping, bloating, indigestion, constipation, or feeling like your food just sits in your stomach like a rock for hours, odds are great that your stomach is not acidic enough. Therefore, when you start to use HCL (starting with the low dose of only one capsule per meal), it's possible to experience heartburn symptoms. This is because you have now added enough HCL to feel that acid when it refluxes back up, but not enough HCL to trigger the LES valve to close properly. Those who continue to increase their HCL dosage until they reach a full dose of 5 capsules per meal will often see these heartburn symptoms disappear once the stomach becomes acidic enough to trigger the valve to close. When the LES valve closes, it blocks the reflux from coming back up.

Some individuals find faster relief by implementing one or more of the following tricks;

1. Eating a dill pickle or two at the end of each meal is often enough to acidify the stomach to a level that will trigger the valve to close.
2. Taking 1000mg of Vitamin C as ascorbic acid before each meal may be enough to boost the HCL you are currently using.
3. In severe cases, taking a few doses of d-limonene before continuing with the HCL protocol may be an effective step for some individuals. Gasses can cause our food to push back up the esophagus. By wiping out a good layer of bacteria in your stomach, you can reduce the amount of gasses being created by that bacteria, therefore reducing the amount of pressure those gasses can create.

Any of these three steps may also allow you to reduce the number of HCL capsules that are required each meal. The d-limonene is a much more aggressive step, so if the dill pickles or ascorbic acid capsules are enough to cease any reflux symptoms, I prefer to see someone go the more gentle route.

When first starting HCL, it is also important to make sure you are not eating starches or sugars with any meal where you will be supplementing HCL capsules. Those carbs can activate the bacteria in your stomach and create more gasses. Once you get up to a full dose of HCL or are able to acidify the stomach enough to trigger the LES valve to close, you should be able to re-introduce higher carb foods while using HCL.

I just started HCL and it makes me nauseous or creates stomach discomfort. Does that mean I don't need to supplement HCL?

It seems that those who need HCL the most, are the same folks who experience some type of discomfort when starting HCL supplementation. In most cases where an individual is making plenty of their own HCL, adding additional HCL will either create a loose stool issue, or a warming-type of discomfort in the stomach. Unfortunately, when people read this and then experience discomfort when starting HCL, they often assume they must not need to add additional HCL since it created such discomfort. Most commonly this seems to occur because these individuals have a bacterial overgrowth in the stomach. The waste from this bacteria creates an alkaline environment in the stomach. When you add HCL to an overly alkaline environment, the reaction of the acid meeting the alkaline waste can create a fizzy mess.

Think about that science fair project volcano where the "lava" starts to bubble and expand and rise out of the top of the volcano. This reaction is caused by acid (vinegar) meeting alkaline (baking soda). This is similar to the reaction that is going on in your stomach if you add HCL to an alkaline environment. That discomfort doesn't mean you don't need HCL. It simply means that you might need to wipe out a good layer of that bacteria before you can use HCL comfortably.

Further acidifying the stomach with dill pickles or ascorbic acid, or taking steps to reduce a bacterial infection in the stomach (like using d-limonene for a week or two), will often allow individuals to start their HCL protocol without the discomfort that was coming from the bubbling mess that was taking place in their stomachs.

What if I am even more constipated after starting Beet Flow and HCL?

For some, Beet Flow can thin the bile pretty quickly and improve bile flow. Remember, bile is the alkaline side of digestion and, in most cases, the more alkaline the stool, the slower it will move. Therefore, if you've improved bile flow, but you have not yet ramped up to a full dose of HCL, your constipation could get worse.

Keep in mind that even if you've ramped up to a full dose of HCL, but your stomach is too alkaline from a bacterial overgrowth, it could still take more time to improve the acidification side of the digestive process. It's not that the supplements "made you more constipated." It's just that you have improved the alkaline side faster than the acid side so your stool has slowed down even further. Once the acidification process improves as much as your bile flow has, the constipation will likely improve. Individuals are often looking for a supplement that will fix their problems. The truth is, it's the correct application of knowledge that primarily fixes problems. Success with supplements comes after and because of the knowledge.

Since I started drinking more water, I'm very tired and/or depressed.

Check your blood pressure at least two hours after a meal. Drinking more water can be very helpful when it comes to improving constipation. However, if your mineral levels are low, you may not qualify to add more water. You may be washing out too many minerals and dropping your blood pressure too low. A lack of minerals is one of the most common contributors to depression. You may need to work more on improving digestion and taking steps to lift your mineral resources before you can increase your water intake.

I've been taking a full dose of HCL but I'm still bloated and constipated.

If you've been at a full dose of HCL for a few weeks and you're still not seeing any improvement to bloating or constipation, you may be dealing with a bacterial infection in your stomach (like George Clooney in our case study earlier in this chapter). Waste from bacteria is alkaline and can make the stomach environment more suitable for the bacteria to thrive. If your stomach is very alkaline and neutralizing the HCL that you are supplementing, five HCL capsules may be only as effective as one or two. This does not mean that you should take fifteen HCL capsules to make up for the alkaline environment. That is not advised. We do, however, see people improve this situation by taking a wider variety of steps to acidify the stomach, or by taking steps to wipe out a good layer of that bacteria, making it easier to acidify the stomach properly. If you're not already eating a dill pickle or two at the end of each meal, and/or taking 1000mg of ascorbic acid before each meal, these steps may be best to try first. If those more gentle steps have no effect for you, d-limonene seems to work well for many when there is a bacterial overgrowth in the stomach. One dose every other morning has been shown to bring improvement for many over a seven to fourteen day period.

I don't recommend taking d-limonene over a long period of time. It can be very pro-catabolic, and seems to be used best in short intervals.

Referencing These FAQs

Don't forget to come back to this chapter and review these case studies and FAQs if you run into any trouble or don't see the results you want to see. Please keep in mind that these are simply real-world examples of steps that have worked for people in specific situations. You still need to monitor your chemistry and apply the steps that are appropriate for you and your biological individuality. By now you understand that just because something worked for one person, that doesn't mean it's going to work for you. Following your numbers and your digestive clues brings in an analytical component and can guide you down the path that should bring you the best results.

If any questions come up that were not covered in this book, don't forget to ask them in our free and private Facebook support group. You can join for free here:
https://www.facebook.com/groups/kickyourfatsupport/

Wha'd He Say?

In this chapter, you learned:

- There's more than one George Clooney.
- Eating too many starches or sugars can exacerbate an Anabolic Imbalance and magnify a chronic constipation issue.
- Drinking more water can often be helpful when attempting to improve constipation, but not every constipated person needs to drink more water. Some individuals simply need to help their body adjust where that water is being sent. Others still may not qualify to increase water intake until they have taken steps to lift their mineral levels.
- Taking Vitamin C as ascorbic acid before meals may help boost the acidifying effects of HCL supplementation and allow an individual to reduce the number of HCL capsules needed to properly acidify the stomach at mealtime.
- If you feel bloated after a meal (maybe you forgot to take your HCL), eating a dill pickle or two is often enough to help acidify the stomach and sooth that distress.

Chapter Twelve (The Sum Up)

Review & Make Your Plan

Now What?

Let's take a moment to lay out the important points that I've covered so you have an easy reference you can use to put your plan together. I know this was a lot of information and you may feel a little overwhelmed and excited at the same time. Just take a deep breath and I'll cover the important points that you don't want to forget and a few that will help you move forward and avoid pitfalls.

You've learned an incredible amount of information so this section is where I pull a Mr. Miyagi and help you put it all together in a usable format. By the end of this wrap-up, you should be saying, "Ah, that's why that bastard had me painting his fence."

Bring It All Together

Achieving lasting relief from constipation is about understanding what is causing *your* constipation. Correcting any digestive issues or imbalances will greatly speed up your results.

Here are major points to remember:

1. Correct any digestive issues so you can pull needed resources out of the food you're eating. DON'T SKIP THIS. If you are not producing enough stomach acid, your stool can move slowly no matter what you do.

2. If an Anabolic Imbalance showed up on your Imbalance Guide, this needs to be addressed in order to see any lasting relief.
3. Increase your water intake so more water can be sent to your bowels. If your blood pressure is low, or if an Electrolyte Deficiency Imbalance appears to be present, be sure to increase your mineral content before increasing water intake. Using concentrated mineral drops in your drinking water may allow you to increase water intake without further lowering blood pressure. Be sure to monitor your blood pressure to know what is right for you.
4. Eat real food! Most processed foods are packed with chemicals, sugars, and carbohydrates that can exacerbate an Anabolic Imbalance. Eating real food also means you need to have more than one meal per day, and don't skip breakfast.
5. If you become extremely plugged up, a teaspoon of epsom salt mixed into an 8-ounce glass of water in the morning can push an individual more catabolic and send more water to the bowels, loosening up the stool. (This is not something I would do on a regular basis, but can be helpful in an <u>urgent</u> situation.)
6. Beyond using Beet Flow and HCL to improve digestion, Vitamin C, as ascorbic acid, will likely be the most successfully used supplement by many of those reading this book (unless your urine pH is already below 5.5). With its ability to further acidify the stool, ascorbic acid can help some people see faster results while they work to improve digestive issues and any imbalances that showed up while self-testing.
7. If you find it difficult to lower urine pH with a strong Anabolic Imbalance, you may need to reduce your starch and sugar intake. Remember, both starches and sugars can have a pro-anabolic effect on many people.

These are some of the most important steps for lasting relief from constipation. Since you have read this book, measured where your chemistry is, and understand how to monitor yourself, you know which of the foregoing factors apply to you the most. Since everyone is different, some of the points may not be as important or even apply to you. Remember, this book is about figuring out your specific body chemistry. It isn't about reading a bunch of stuff and then just following the summary list at the end. It's about responding to measurements. You can't manage what you don't measure. Pay attention to your progress and make adjustments accordingly.

Fix Digestive Issues

By reviewing your *Digestive Issue Validators* on your *Imbalance Guide*, you know if you need to put some attention toward improving digestion. Odds are great that if you're reading this book, you do. **Don't skip this step. You will not get the results you want if you don't improve digestion through supplementation.** I have seen people improve imbalances using only food and lifestyle choices; but very few will correct digestive issues without the aid of supplements, at least temporarily. If you're not digesting food successfully, and your body is not getting the resources it needs, producing enough HCL to keep your stool moving will be difficult. Digestion is huge. Don't skip it.

Correct Your Imbalances

Taking steps toward correcting an imbalance and *actually* correcting an imbalance are not the same thing. To Improve symptoms requires correcting the imbalance that is causing those symptoms. If you take steps to correct an Electrolyte Deficiency Imbalance, but your blood pressure is still incredibly low and all your numbers are still pointing to an Electrolyte Deficiency Imbalance, then more needs to be done to correct the issue.

You don't want to be the guy who says, "I did what you told me to do and I still can't poop." Put more stock in your numbers than in what you are doing to correct them. If your self-test numbers still show an imbalance, the symptoms will often still be there to go right along with that imbalance. Just because you did some work to correct the imbalance doesn't mean that you did ENOUGH work to correct YOUR imbalance. For some, it will take more effort and more time to see the results and move the body closer to balance. If you are experiencing a stubborn imbalance, get help from a professional who can guide you or see if anyone in our free support group has any suggestions. You're probably just missing a key point or doing things to work against yourself as you try to create improvements.

Monitor Your Numbers

Monitoring is a crucial step. When a person starts feeling better, it becomes easy to forget why this improvement came to be. I see a lot of clients who do the work to see improvement and then they stop doing the right things, go back to their old habits, and wonder why they're sitting on the toilet without any action again. You wouldn't workout for one month, lose a little weight and expect that weight to continue to stay off if you stopped working out. You have to continue to be aware of how your body is operating if you want to continue to see results. Yes, the amount of monitoring you'll need to do may drastically decrease once the body is in balance. Monitoring less frequently will certainly be appropriate once you're feeling great. But you still need to check your numbers from time to time and make sure everything is going as planned. This will allow you to steer clear of many problems.

Don't Work Against Yourself

Taking steps in the right direction is absolutely the most important way to get started. However, the steps you take in the wrong direction still count. If you're dealing with an Anabolic Imbalance, continuing to eat a lot of sugar or starches can still exacerbate that imbalance and make your constipation worse.

Don't forget that you now have the tools to correct the cravings that cause you to eat all that junk. By correcting those cravings, reducing starches and sugars becomes a lot easier.

Try to remember that there is already a lot working against you, and it is likely not your fault that you are dealing with these issues. I feel like some of the despicable farming methods used in this country have to be responsible for a lot of our deficiencies. You may feel people shouldn't have to work this hard at living, and you're right; but profiteering in the farming industry is a reality. Keep this in the back of your mind in case your issues return, so you can become vigilant again about taking the right steps. In the same way that it can be fun to grow a nice plant, it can also be enjoyable to continue feeling better and having more vitality.

Make Your Plan

If you fail to plan, you plan to fail. Is it a little annoying that I said that? Yes, it is. But if it gets you to put together a course of action, I'm okay with being annoying. It doesn't take much for life to get in the way. The good news is that any time your stool starts to get too hard, you can use that as a reminder that you have yet to take the time to make the needed improvements. Writing up a plan in a notebook can help you avoid that reminder.

Since what you eat counts, know what you're going to eat before it's time to eat. If you wait until you're starving to decide what you're going to eat that day, you're going to end up with a scoop of Golden Grahams in a taco shell. Once major hunger strikes, all proper judgment can go out the window. Plan what you're going to eat ahead of time and you will make better choices.

In a similar vein, grocery stores have a magic threshold that erases your brain as you walk in the sliding glass doors. Know what you're going to buy before you get to the store.

If you find that you need to use supplements to improve digestion or an imbalance, plan that as well. Most of us live our lives on the go. Burger King doesn't carry the supplements you need, so you can't just drive through and grab them while you're out. Success will take making some new habits; but when you plan ahead, everything gets easier.

You're not going to make just one plan and stick with that forever. Remember that your plan will be adjusted as the measurements change on your *Data Tracking Sheet*.

Avoid Screwing Yourself Over

There really is no such thing as a "side effect"—only direct effects. When you use a supplement or change your diet, or increase or decrease water intake... all these things have the ability to change your body chemistry, and that change can create an effect. It's not a side effect; you did something and things changed. It's a direct effect.

I have heard "side effect" described as choosing to put up with poisonous or negative effects in order to have a particular benefit. Don't you think the better choice is to have only benefit? Let's choose the positive without the price of a negative.

Avoid looking at these changes like, "This doesn't work for me," and therefore quit trying to balance your body. Whatever change you are creating is just more information. If something creates the opposite reaction than what you're looking for, then you can use that information to steer in the right direction. If you understand how to look at the clues, you don't have to jump ship just because a bird crapped on the deck of the boat.

If you choose a course of action, and your measurements show things going in the opposite direction, try to remember that a change in measurement that goes in the opposite direction is still wonderful information. You're finding your way. If a supplement or food choice doesn't work, that information can go a long way in determining what WILL work for you. Why did a choice push you in the opposite direction? Use that information to look for an answer. Find a practitioner to help you decipher why anything might push you in the wrong direction. If you need help but can't afford it, join the free community described below, and post questions to see if other community members have experience with similar situations.

Here are two examples. A young man by the name of Soupy was having stomach pains. (Good thing I changed his name for this book. That would have been very unfortunate if his name was really Soupy.) Soupy's body was not creating enough stomach acid to break down the food he was eating. As his food would rot and ferment, gases were created that would expand his stomach and cause pain and bloating. He started using HCL supplements and immediately his pain began to reduce. But he also started experiencing painful heartburn.

Remember, the LES (Lower Esophageal Sphincter) valve at the bottom of the esophagus is triggered to close when stomach acid levels rise due to digestion kicking in. Without enough stomach acid, that valve doesn't close and you can have reflux. If there is no stomach acid, you won't even feel that reflux because there is no acid coming up to burn you (you can learn more about this in Appendix A, or by listening to our *Kick It Naturally* episode, *Understanding Acid Reflux, Heartburn and GERD*). If you begin to add HCL supplementation, now you have some acid in your stomach. But if you haven't reached a high enough dose to trigger that valve to close, now you have reflux that contains acid and you get burned. This can happen even if you are avoiding starches while you initially begin increasing HCL intake (as explained in chapter three.)

Soupy thought that since he had never experienced heartburn before, it must be the HCL that was giving him heartburn so he stopped using it. If he had just increased his dosage according to instructions, his acid levels would have triggered the valve to close, reflux would have stopped and he could have continued receiving the relief from his stomach pains that follow every meal for him. By misunderstanding what his body was telling him, he missed an opportunity to improve his health and eliminate a horrible discomfort he lives with every day.

Another example is what happened to Sugarplum. Yes, her name really is Sugarplum. Sugarplum wanted to correct her Electrolyte Deficiency Imbalance and also lose weight. She began using supplements to improve her imbalance and correct her digestion. She lowered her carb intake so her insulin would not spike as often and cause her body to store fat. This helped her to drop weight.

But her cravings for sugar also began to skyrocket. She had never had uncontrollable cravings before so she assumed that the supplements she was using had messed up her body in some way and caused her to be a sugar freak so she stopped taking supplements. This is a fun deduction; but, as an option, we could also use science and logic to figure out what happened to Sugarplum.

You learned earlier that cravings are mostly created from low minerals and/or low blood sugar. Sugarplum was taking the right steps to improve her Electrolyte Deficiency Imbalance but her imbalance was strong and her blood pressure was still extremely low, indicating that she still had a low level of minerals in her system. Once she lowered her carb and sugar intake to lose weight, there was now nothing left to buffer the system—not enough minerals and not enough sugars. Cravings almost always skyrocket when sugars and minerals are both low.

Before she started attempting to raise her mineral levels with supplements, she never had cravings because she was buffering her system with carbs and sugars (which is the reason she had gained weight in the first place). As long as sugars are high, a person won't get those cravings. Weight gain often shows up as a result of keeping those sugars high, but the uncontrollable cravings can be kept at bay.

If Sugarplum would have added some medium-carb foods (not starch) to her diet, instead of eliminating all carbs, the sugars from those carbs could have continued to buffer her low mineral content. Her weight loss would have been more gradual, but that's okay since she would also be keeping her cravings away. As her mineral content and blood pressure began to climb, she could have reduced her carbs further at that point if she still needed to lose weight. The important lesson here is not to look at the changes you make as "not working" or "causing crazy side effects." As I said, these were all direct effects—not side effects. These effects just needed to be looked at logically so she could use them to steer her next move.

The moral of both these examples is this: Don't screw yourself. Most people never have an opportunity to correct the issues that are plaguing them. Don't screw yourself out of that opportunity because you decide to ignore how your system works. Listen to the clues that show up. If they don't make sense to you, get help from someone who can help you decipher them. Stay determined and keep in mind why you started this journey. You can kick your constipation naturally if you're willing to do the work and stick with it. Do self-tests. Measure your numbers so your situation will make sense to you. Then, you can regulate what is needed.

Finding Supplements

Remember, a lot of the supplements I talk about in this book will not be found in stores. Most products that I talk about in this book can be found on www.NaturalReference.com. Don't forget about digestion when ordering supplements. If you're like most of the readers of this book, digestion will be the priority and you will likely be ordering Betaine HCL, Beet Flow, Digesti-zyme, and pH strips to cover all three aspects of digestion and to monitor your progress. All of these products are available without a health coach.

Optimal Measurement Ranges

Optimal pHs According To Breath Rate

Breath Rate	Urine pH	Saliva pH
Above 16	5.8 - 6.3	6.5 - 7.0
Below 16	5.5 - 6.0	6.5 - 7.0

Optimal Blood Pressure Reading
120/80
A systolic number between 112 and 130 is considered to be in range.
A diastolic number between 74 and 87 is considered to be in range.

Optimal Breath Rate
Between 14-18 breaths per minute

Optimal Breath Hold Time
Between 41 - 64 seconds

Continue To Learn

Just like anything, the more you learn, the easier it becomes not to suck at it. Continue learning. Visit our website at www.KickItInNaturally.com and soak in piles of free information. Type any keyword in the search box to see if we've covered that topic in a podcast, article or video.

What Else Are You Struggling With?

If you have other health issues you are hoping to improve, I would love to hear from you. Simply go to www.KickItNaturally.com and click on "Contact Us" and send me a message.

I can't legally give you one-on-one advice, but when I hear the issues that people need help improving, and the things that haven't worked for them, it can really help us figure out what type of content we should be working on next, or what topics we should be covering on our next show.

If we've already made some content that might help you, I'll even try to send you a link so you can get your answers much quicker than it took me to find my own.

Follow Me

Join more than 230,000 fans and follow us on Facebook. Click on "Like" and then hover over that button to click on "Get Notifications." Otherwise, Facebook only shares page posts with a fraction of the page's followers and you may miss out on big announcements.

Facebook.com/KickItInTheNuts
Facebook.com/KickItNaturally
Twitter - @KickItInTheNuts

Our Radio Show

This is fun. Be sure you follow us on Facebook and we will post topics every week for our upcoming shows. You can add your questions to our posts and we'll cover them for you on the show. It's almost like you're there, but I don't need to bring extra chairs into the studio. My co-hosts are Kinna McInroe and Will Wolfgang Schmidt. Kinna was the little red-head, Nina, in the movie *Office Space*. She's lost over a hundred pounds with me since then and she is a riot. Will is a celebrity trainer who works with just about every fancy person on the planet. We have a great time and I think we accidentally teach things.

To browse a wide variety of topics we've covered on previous shows, go to www.learn.kickitnaturally.com/full-list-of-show-topics/

Give Yourself A Reminder

Once you begin to feel better, it's pretty easy to forget what you've learned and slip back into old habits. It's hard to remind ourselves to occasionally review the things we've learned, even if those things have changed our lives for the better. Many readers have reported benefiting from subscribing to our free content. When you subscribe to our free podcast on iTunes or Stitcher (for Android), or to our free Youtube channel, you'll get free weekly content. When you swing by Youtube, or open the podcast app on your phone, new shows will remind you to check in and learn something new or get a reminder of the things that have helped.

To subscribe on iTunes or Stitcher, download either free app to your phone, search for Kick It Naturally, and click on subscribe. It's all free.

You can also subscribe to our Youtube channel and keep up with our latest videos here: www.youtube.com/c/KickItNaturally

Help Us Spread the Word or Become a Coach

How annoyed are you that it has taken this long to find this information? Once I got over being angry, I knew I wanted to share this info with anyone I could. The best ways to help us spread the word are to subscribe to our podcast, leave us a review on iTunes, and leave a review for this book on Amazon. Those steps increase our rankings so more people can find us. If you want to reach more people that you know, follow us on Facebook and share our posts so your friends can happen upon this information just like you did.

If you want to take things to the next level and become a health coach, check out our online health pro course at www.HealthProCourse.com. With nearly 300 videos, we walk you through the process of learning how to look at other people's physiology, start your own career as a health coach, or just learn more so you can help your loved ones improve their health.

Join The Community And Get Support

Join the free and private Facebook group found here:
www.facebook.com/groups/kickyourfatsupport/
It started as a weight loss support group, but has evolved into a place where people come to ask questions about all sorts of health issues. Just click on "Join Group" in the upper right hand corner. Make friends, share goals and successes and find answers to your questions from people who are going through the same journey. Everything posted in the group is visible only to others in the group. Therefore, you can post things like, "I just pooped my pants again. Any suggestions?" and you don't have to worry about broadcasting that to all of Facebook.

Be Excited

Right now, in your hand, you are holding answers that some people search for their entire lives and never find. You now have knowledge that can be the "cheat sheet" to your health and your life. Don't take it for granted.

Final Words

For the final words of this book, I select thimble and orange marmalade.

APPENDIX A

More Digestive Explanations

Reflux, Heartburn And GERD

Now that you understand the benefits of both acid production and bile flow working correctly, let's talk about issues that can pop up when one side is not working optimally. I'm referring to the fiction that is the billion dollar industry of reflux, heartburn, and GERD (gastroesophageal reflux disease). The marketing surrounding these issues may mislead an individual more than just about any other current health information out there. First of all, there are many different causes of reflux; but very few cases, if any, are actually caused by "too much acid," as advertisers explain when marketing their products.

At the bottom of your esophagus, there is a little valve called an LES, or lower esophageal sphincter. This valve opens to let food enter the stomach and then it closes, so that the food doesn't go back up your esophagus and burn you. Sometimes, people have a small hiatal hernia where part of the stomach is pulled up above the diaphragm. This can keep that valve from closing and can result in an acid reflux problem. That is one possibility.

However, the most common cause of reflux problems involves the acid level of the stomach. The LES is actually HCL sensitive, meaning that when the stomach makes enough HCL, it activates that valve to close so digesting food doesn't reflux back up. I've already mentioned that some people don't make enough HCL on their own. So doesn't it make sense that, if there isn't enough HCL in the stomach to trigger the valve, the valve would stay open and they would get reflux? People aren't having reflux because of too much acid; they're having reflux because there is not enough acid.

Pharmaceutical companies sell us drugs that turn the acid off, so that when we experience reflux, we can't feel the burning and we assume the originating issue has been dealt with. The problem with that is twofold. First, the stomach also contains digestive enzymes that can come back up with reflux. These digestive enzymes are made to break down protein. What is the esophagus made of? Yes, protein. Therefore, using these drugs stops the burning sensation, but it doesn't stop all the damage that reflux can cause. A reduction in acid coming up could certainly reduce damage. However, it's important to understand that the enzymes coming back up the esophagus still have the ability to cause damage as well. The second problem created by turning off the acid is... you just turned off the acid. I've already covered how important your stomach acid is, how it is the defense barrier for your entire body and how it's an ignorant idea to turn it off.

When you hear about a drug being a proton pump inhibitor (PPI), this refers to the hydrogen proton pump in the human body. These drugs restrict the body from producing hydrogen. Hydrogen is required for the body to make its own HCL, so by turning off the hydrogen, you turn off the acid. Not only are the proton-pump-inhibitor-type drugs another punch in the mouth to your liver (I already discussed how all drugs work by overwhelming the liver enough to be able to stay in the system and do their job), they also turn off your digestion. Now, any food you eat not only doesn't nourish your body like it is intended to, but also this undigested, rotting, fermenting food becomes another problem for your body to try to remove or to store in fat cells. Pretty good little pill, huh?

To reduce reflux, most reflux sufferers can actually *increase* the amount of stomach acid they have which will trigger the LES to close so they no longer experience reflux. This also allows the body to fully break down its food, pull out the minerals and then use those minerals to make the proper amount of stomach acid. Remember to follow the guidelines in chapter three on implementing HCL supplementation. It's important to start slow and ramp up your dose. In the beginning, It can also be crucial to avoid starches and sugars with any meal where you are supplementing with HCL. Those carbohydrates have the ability to excite bacteria, causing more gasses and more pressure to push food back up the esophagus. Once you have corrected the reflux issue, you may be able to add starches and sugars back into meals that include HCL supplementation.

To learn more about how to improve these issues, go to www.KickItNaturally.com and search for reflux in the search box. There, you'll find our podcast episode on Acid Reflux, Heartburn, and GERD.

Crohn's, Colitis, And IBS

What about the other end of digestion? What about the bile side of the action? If bile is not flowing well enough to neutralize the acid product coming from the stomach, now there is acid going through the intestines. And why does the stomach make acid? The primary job of stomach acid is to help digest protein. It's the hydrochloric acid that breaks down food and allows protein to become accessible to the body. Think about it; if you don't neutralize that acid, what do you think it's going to do to your intestines? Your intestines are made out of protein, just like your esophagus. How about that? Does anybody you know have symptoms that were diagnosed as IBS, Crohn's, or colitis? Don't you think this could just be the acid that has been produced in the stomach, that has not been neutralized sufficiently in the duodenum by the proper amount of alkaline bile? Now this acid product goes through the intestines like "Zingo!" Why? Because the acidity of this product is making the intestines burn and the body is going to respond to this acidity and march that product right through the person in a big damn hurry. With this understanding, doesn't it make sense that it comes shooting out the back door in such a rush?

Beyond that, sodium likes to follow chloride. Water likes to follow sodium. So there's also going to be sodium that is attracted to this chloride in the hydrochloric acid (the hydrochloric acid that didn't get neutralized). Then more water will go to the bowels since chloride from HCL that has not been neutralized will draw the sodium with its water into the bowel. It would be like the boy band One Direction showing up to your cookout because they wanted hot dogs. Not only would you have five less hot dogs, you would also have a yard filled with thousands of screaming little girls. The good news is, the water rushing to this guy's bowels will help dilute this acid product that is burning the intestinal walls. The bad news is, he just crapped his pants. This guy is going to have diarrhea and he is going to wonder why, when he sits on the john, it's like he was shot from rockets. It's because his body is saying, "Get this acid product that is burning the daylights out of my little intestines out of here!"

Probiotics and gut flora are a hot topic these days. The people who experience these diarrhea-type issues need help in this arena because that un-neutralized acid scorching through their intestines just fried their gut flora. The terrain needs to be right for gut flora to flourish. As you can imagine, the towering inferno from hell is not the right terrain. This is a very vague explanation, but it's a great visualization to help explain the balance that is required in order for digestion to function correctly. Both ends of the process are important. It's clear that trouble arises when one side or the other isn't holding up its end of the bargain. To learn more, go to www.KickItNaturally.com and search for Crohn's, colitis, or IBS.

Birth Control Medications

Many birth control medications contain synthetic estrogen. It appears that synthetic estrogen has the ability to sludge up bile, therefore restricting proper bile flow. The liver is made to excrete all the estrogen that a woman produces each day. When a liver is overwhelmed and not functioning properly, estrogen excretion may not be optimal and the woman can become estrogen dominant. Therefore, the level at which excess synthetic estrogen may sludge up the bile can vary greatly from woman to woman, depending on her liver function. In any case, bile that is too thick and sticky can't flow correctly, and I've already covered how bad that is.

When bile can't flow correctly, you can't properly digest your food and break it down into its elemental components. You may also get nauseous because bile is the main method that the body uses to remove toxins out the south gate (bowels). If your bile flow reduces because of birth control meds, those toxins can build up and you can experience nausea. It's your body's way of telling you, "Look, we can't handle the food you've put in here, do you really need to keep adding more?"

In addition to turning off the body's main path of junk removal, birth control medications are a synthetic drug. In order for the dose to stay in the body long enough to do its job, it has to be a dose high enough to overwhelm the liver. Otherwise, the liver would just remove it from the body before the drug had a chance to perform its intended purpose. So, any drug can't work unless it first punches your liver in the mouth. Now, the drug occupies the liver and the liver can't do its normal job of removing toxins, or properly removing estrogen. As the toxins get backed up, you get nauseous or you can gain weight since your body is forced to store those toxins in fat cells. That's one of the reasons so many women gain weight on the pill. If a birth control drug overwhelms the liver, reducing the ability of the liver to remove extra estrogen that was contained in that drug, that could result in the bile thickening more and more as time passes. The thicker the bile gets, the less it has the ability to flow correctly, and the harder it is for the liver to do its job and this cycle could continue to snowball.

Birth control meds are also believed to kill all, or most of, your intestinal flora. If birth control medication stops a woman's bile from flowing correctly, there is nothing to cool off the acid product coming from the stomach and the intestinal flora can burn up. Without the beneficial bacteria, bad guys start to take over, creating an overgrowth of harmful bacteria and yeast, like candida.

Just in case you didn't catch my drift here, birth control medication can be one of the worst things a woman can do if she wants to have a healthy body. I realize pregnancy has the potential to wreak havoc on the body as well; at least with pregnancy, 10 years later you have someone to take out your trash for you. However, there is a freedom of choice in these matters, and there are birth control options available that will allow you to continue digesting your food properly.

Gallbladder Removal / Gallstones / Olive Oil-Lemon Drink

When I see a client with health issue after health issue, one of my first questions is, "Do you still have your gallbladder?" Doctors are taught that the gallbladder really doesn't do anything anyway; so, if there are stones or blockages, why not just yank it out? The problem is that your gallbladder is where your body stores bile, and without the proper amount of bile, you can't digest your food completely. The gallbladder also concentrates the bile, so that when its alkalinity drops down on the acid product from the stomach, there is a good digestive sizzle. You've already learned how proper digestion is needed to obtain nutrients from your food. Eventually, without proper digestion, all the mineral and nutrient deficiencies will cause problems and even imbalances. The majority of health issues lead back to digestion in one way or another. You can digest food correctly only if you have enough acid in your stomach, enough bile from the gallbladder, and bicarb and enzymes from the pancreas dropping down into your duodenum. Without a gallbladder there is no bile storage, so you rarely have enough bile.

The digestive system is a crazy, complex, miraculous machine. With so many bits and pieces at play, the system is vulnerable to problems that would cause it to function below par. Do you really think a system will work the way it is meant to if you take out part of it (i.e. the gallbladder) and chuck it in the garbage? When any part of the digestive process is not functioning, troubles can show up for months, decades, or even a lifetime. You may not even know you're having digestive concerns because you feel okay when you eat (or you've forgotten what it feels like to feel good). But the lack of nutrients coming into the system, which can be created by a lack of digestion, is always going to come back to bite you in the butt. They may even literally bite you in the butt. (That was a parasite joke for those who didn't keep up.)

There is one technique that can simulate bile production from the gallbladder. Many people who have lost their gallbladder use this technique with success to improve their digestion. You can buy ox bile supplements in most health food stores. However, remember that bile is alkaline. If you take an ox bile product with your food, you're going to neutralize your stomach acid while it's still in your stomach. That's not fun and will likely make you feel very bloated. The trick is to take the ox bile product about two hours after a meal, or at least an hour before a meal. I like the hour before a meal best, but it can be difficult to remember that all the time. By moving that bile through your intestines between your meals, you can neutralize the acid product coming from your stomach and almost simulate the sizzle that all the cool kids have in their digestion. This ox bile really isn't going to work as well as true digestion, but without a gallbladder, this ox bile schedule can be one of the most effective options for any type of improvement.

Many people who have had their gallbladder removed will eventually end up with some type of loose stool issue. Since there isn't enough bile storage to neutralize the acid coming from the stomach, that acid just keeps trucking through the intestinal tract. The hitch is that this issue usually arises months or even years after they've had their gallbladder removed, so they never connect the two events. Using an ox bile product (as I described in the previous paragraph) is the most effective method I know to improve or prevent these loose stool issues, outside of buying a used gallbladder from someone at a garage sale (though I'm not sure how that would work with all the haggling that goes on at garage sales).

If you have gallstones and you're thinking about having your gallbladder removed, you might want to try smashing yourself in the face with a hammer instead. You may indeed prefer a nice hammer smashing over some of the troubles I have seen from people who have had their gallbladder removed. There are things you can do to improve your gallbladder function and help soften those gallstones without cutting out the whole package. If someone told you that your big toe needed to be removed, you would make sure he knew what he was talking about; you would also be careful that you did not get a "second opinion" from some crony of the guy who gave you the first opinion. We know that because of gangrene or something very grievous, some big toes do need to be removed. But if you went into the doctor's office with toenail fungus and the doctor said the answer was to cut off your toe, you would probably find somebody else to help you. It seems a person would value his gallbladder at least as much as his big toe. I think internal organs generally eclipse appendages in value, but that's just me. If doctors were educated on how digestion really works, it would eliminate the billion dollar industry of antacids and acid-stopping drugs. Since doctors are not educated on how digestion works, doesn't it make sense that they view the gallbladder as if it were a disposable Ziploc baggie that can just be dumped in the trash?

There is an old-school remedy for a gallbladder attack that still holds true today. Instructions were even printed right on the label of every carton of epsom salt. The label said, "Take 4 tsp of epsom salt mixed in warm water." This will clear most gallbladder attacks because it can squirt the bile through and clear out the blockage. Be warned that this little trick can give you some crazy diarrhea since epsom salt is magnesium sulfate. Both magnesium and sulfur products can push more water to the bowels, so a large dose of magnesium sulfate can create a bit of a show shooting out the back door. But an episode of diarrhea beats a lifetime of diarrhea every time. You would still need to do the work to get your bile to flow better so you can soften up those stones and keep more stones from forming, but this is a great little trick that has worked for over a hundred years for those suffering from gallbladder attacks.

There are some great recipes on the Internet for olive oil and lemon drinks that can help clear out a gallbladder. However, if you do any cleanses like this that can also clear out a liver, and your bile isn't flowing well, you're just dumping all these toxins into the body while the body has no way to remove them. This can trigger some crazy rashes as a result of the body trying to push junk out through the skin, or you can really overload and hurt your kidneys as they try to handle the whole load. With this in mind, be sure you learn how to thin your bile and get it flowing better with specific beet leaf products before you try any of those liver/gallbladder-type cleanses. They can bring about some big trouble if you don't. Are you listening to me right now? This is important, so please don't ignore what I'm saying and go straight for a heavy duty liver cleanse without first addressing your bile flow with the beet leaf products described in chapter three.

H. Pylori Infections & Natural Protocols

In the world of research, it is commonly assumed that the decline in HCL production observed through later adult life (approximately 30% of the population over 65 years old doesn't make enough HCL) is a "normal" and common consequence of getting older. However, recent studies indicate that the secretion of HCL does not decrease in the stomach as a person ages; HCL production actually appears to increase, especially in men. Even more evidence shows that the frequently observed reduction or loss of HCL production is generally the result of asymptomatic infections. The most common infection of this type for humans is Helicobacter pylori, or I'll just say H. pylori like all the fancy people say.

It is now a popular opinion that the older you are, the better your chances that you currently have an H. pylori infection. That percentage even goes up with each year of life that you have under your belt. For example, a 40-year-old person would have a 40% chance of having an H. pylori infection. I'm not a fan of treating according to the "at your age you need…" point of view, but these numbers do give a good indication of how common an H. pylori infection can be.

The chances of an H. pylori infection goes up dramatically if you have ever used any type of acid reflux or heartburn medication that turns off stomach acid. Many believe that it is difficult for H. pylori to colonize in a stomach with sufficient stomach acid; but if that level of stomach acid is temporarily reduced, H. pylori can invade and then find ways to survive once the production of stomach acid returns. It appears that H. pylori have the ability to crawl up into the mucous lining of the stomach, escape the acid during digestion, and then come back out once acid levels have dropped again. I believe that is why, if people with an H. pylori infection begin to use HCL supplementation or other products designed to kill H. pylori, those people will experience some improvement in their reflux symptoms. Yet, they won't experience complete eradication unless they take extra measures.

H. pylori can be such a major factor with digestion because this bacteria eats hydrogen. Hydrogen is what your body uses to mix with chloride to make HCL. If H. pylori is eating all of your hydrogen, your body won't be able to make very much HCL. I discussed earlier how countless people who are not making enough stomach acid likely don't have the minerals needed to make HCL. But you can see how an H. pylori infection could scarf up enough hydrogen to remove the other important factor in HCL production: The hydrogen.

Most of the acid reflux and heartburn medications out there are proton pump inhibitors, or PPIs, as they are called. They work by turning off the proton pump that makes hydrogen. Now the body can't make HCL anymore, so the person doesn't feel the reflux and the symptom is gone, just like I talked about earlier. But these drugs were actually developed to take care of H. pylori. By turning off hydrogen, you can starve H. pylori and they die. It just turned out that scientists realized turning off HCL production (and therefore digestion) could remove the symptoms of any reflux or heartburn, so they began marketing PPI products in that manner.

The compelling detail about these PPI drugs is that they can starve H. pylori, yet your odds of having an H. pylori infection increase if you've ever used one of these drugs. How could that be? Since you asked, I guess I'll tell you. It is widely accepted that most people won't start making hydrogen again for up to three weeks after they have ceased taking any type of proton pump inhibitor medication. This means people are not making HCL as long as they can't make hydrogen. Consequently, even if the lack of hydrogen starves the H. pylori out of existence, the acid-free "window of opportunity" is open for two or three weeks for any little critters to come in and set up camp. You may recall I talked about how H. pylori can exist in an acid stomach as long as they get in while the acid levels are low. Isn't it realistic that H. pylori could make their way back in while people are barely starting to make hydrogen again? Maybe individuals are making enough hydrogen to feed bacteria, but not enough to create the acid barrier that keeps them all out.

This lack of acid barrier can also allow other types of bacteria in the front door—other bacteria that may live on sugar instead of hydrogen. If these bacteria can flourish in the three-week window of an acid-free environment in the stomach, they can create an alkaline environment which could stay more alkaline even after the body begins making HCL again. The waste product from some bacteria is alkaline, therefore making the environment more inhabitable for them. Do you see how just having the door open can set up the environment for H. pylori to reinfect the body? This isn't even considering the fact that, once you turn some people's digestion off, they have a hard time getting it started again. Seeing that the body can't break down what is being eaten well enough to pull the minerals out of the food, that individual may not have enough minerals needed for the body to make HCL again once the hydrogen turns back on. This shows how easy it can be for people to lose their optimal digestion for weeks, months, or even years. No matter how you chalk it up, you can see the wide variety of circumstances that could allow a bacterial infection to make its way into the body.

You may recall how reflux, or heartburn, is often caused by the activity of bacteria in the stomach. Doctors who deal with this issue a lot often tell me that, when they test for an infection in the stomach, they almost always find H. pylori and maybe some other type of pathogen as well. When symptoms of a bacterial infection in the stomach are present, H. pylori is very commonly at least one of the culprits. Other than creating common digestive symptoms like reflux, heartburn, or decreased ability to digest food, an H. pylori infection could exist for years, or even decades, without showing any real symptoms. Therefore, this infection will very often go undiagnosed. The new DNA stool tests that your doctor can order can be expensive if your insurance doesn't cover them; but it can be nice to know if you have an infection or not. Even without lab tests to confirm the presence of H. pylori, I've seen people just use supplemental products as if they have an infection since most products used to fight H. pylori would be acceptable for temporary use whether you had an infection or not.

Before you become too aggressive towards an H. pylori infection you are not certain exists, it might be best to take steps to improve digestion first. Since you may be dealing with a number of imbalances at first, the extra supplements it can take to wipe out an H. pylori infection could be overwhelming. I like to see someone first add HCL supplementation; additional HCL is usually all that is needed to increase acid production. If HCL capsules do not correct the problem and you feel like you may be dealing with H. pylori infection, using the information described below may be the best bet for you. You could also enlist the help of a professional health coach, as they may be able to better understand some of your numbers and determine if an H. pylori test, or supplement protocol is right for you.

Side note: If a person is dealing with a Sympathetic Imbalance, (maybe they are constantly stressed or living at the speed of light) this stress can also restrict a person's ability to properly produce sufficient HCL. If this sounds familiar, an excellent option may be to simply calm down before you jump to the conclusion that you must have an H. pylori infection.

Here is the complex supplement protocol that seems to be most effective at wiping out an H. pylori infection. This infection can be difficult to take care of. It's my experience that a few things need to be used in conjunction with each other to have a successful outcome. When fighting H. pylori, even the medical world will use two different antibiotics and a proton pump inhibitor at the same time to wipe them out. The problems with this method are: Not only are you using antibiotics which kill bacteria but still lay the foundation for fungal problems later on, you are also turning off the protective acid barrier and opening the door for any bad guys that want to come in while the acid is shut down. I'm not much of a fan for any strategy that lets every annoying little scumbag in the world of bacteria, fungus, and parasites come on in for a party.

Here are the main players in the natural world that seem to get the best results when used together in an attempt to eradicate H. pylori:

Zinc

Zinc has the ability to kill H. pylori, specifically liquid zinc in the form of zinc sulphate. This is a great place to start. A company called BodyBio makes a liquid zinc that I like a lot. I've seen people use 15 drops twice a day with pretty good success. Zinc is also believed to be one of the minerals needed to produce your own HCL, so that can be a nice bonus. If you're using HCL supplementation, including zinc in your protocol may be a good idea because doing so will give your body an additional tool it can use to make its own HCL. Empirical Labs makes a digestive enzyme called Digesti-zyme that includes a little bit of zinc. This is a great formula to use when you're trying to increase HCL production.

Along with zinc, it is also popular to use an amino acid, L-Carnosine, for this issue. You can even find "zinc carnosine" manufactured by many companies. I still like to use the liquid zinc even if I'm going to use zinc carnosine. If I use plain L-Carnosine capsules with the liquid zinc, one L-Carnosine capsule twice a day seems to be effective.

HCL

Since H. pylori are happier in an alkaline environment, increasing stomach acid is always an important step. Not only can H. pylori scarf up all your hydrogen so the body can't make much HCL, they also pee ammonia. Ammonia is an alkaline substance and can alkalize the stomach even further, totally pimping out their pad to optimize life for H. pylori and many other bacteria that would be eradicated in a more acid stomach pH.

Pyloricin

Pyloricin is an herbal product made by a company called Pharmax. It's available to consumers at many health food stores and online retailers. When you open the bottle and smell the capsules, your reaction will be, "Oh yeah, I wouldn't want to live in a place that smelled like that either, so I imagine this will work nicely." It's not disgusting to take, you're just swallowing capsules. But it does make your pee smell funky so you know it's doing something, right? The word on the street (and the words coming out of my mouth from my experience) is that this product works better than just about anything else out there.

I've seen people take two capsules, three times a day, and work through two bottles and be done. I still use this product in conjunction with other efforts I'm describing here since I don't think any of these supplements would do the job on their own. I will also add that if you are a toxic person, and maybe you get nauseous easily, you will want to start slowly on this product because it is strong and could be a little overwhelming to a sensitive person.

d-Limonene

d-Limonene seems to be very effective at seeping into the mucous layer in the stomach and wiping out bacteria. However, it is very pro-catabolic and should be used with caution. Most people do well if they skip a day between doses and use it only once a day, first thing in the morning, when we are intended to be more catabolic. d-Limonene is a natural orange peel extract.

Pepto-Bismol

What? I know, I know. Pepto-Bismol is not very natural. But it's basically just bismuth. Be sure to use the original and not the cherry flavored or any of the other varieties that have extra junk in them. Bismuth is a heavy metal that is found in our bodies already and can be very effective at wiping out bacteria in the stomach. When H. pylori begin to die from the other supplements you are using, they can often clench on to the side of your stomach and create a cramping feeling. It's really not that fun. If you feel this, you can take Pepto-Bismol which will help finish them off and relieve your cramping faster. (Not to be confused with menstrual cramps, this is not the same thing.) The cramping may still last a while longer, but using the Pepto can reduce the duration of those cramps. Since the active ingredient, bismuth, is a heavy metal, I try not to use Pepto-Bismol for longer than a week to ten days at a time.

So, Pepto-Bismol isn't one that I start off with, but I do recommend having it on hand once you start the rest of this protocol so you can be ready if you experience any stomach cramps.

Bee Propolis or Mastic Gum

I describe bee propolis and mastic gum together because they work in similar fashions and seem to be the most popular choice. I've never seen anyone with H. pylori use one of these products without improvement, but I've also never seen anyone totally eradicate the problem with one of these supplements and nothing else. I'll explain how they work and you'll understand why. I do, however, feel that they are an excellent part of the arsenal I would use to wipe out H. pylori. I just hear a lot of people suggesting that this is enough to take care of the problem and I don't agree with that at all.

When a mouse crawls into a beehive, the bees will sting it to death and the mouse invader will be neutralized. Now, if you're a bee, you have a dead and rotting mouse in your house. It's not like the bees can just chuck it out the back door. What they do is cover the mouse in what is called propolis. It basically mummifies the mouse so that it doesn't rot in the hive. That's why bee propolis is used as a natural antibiotic. It goes in and essentially mummifies any bacteria so it can be safely removed from the body. Mastic gum works in the same way. The problem is, these bacteria can crawl up into the mucous lining of the stomach and avoid being swept away in a sticky cocoon. I certainly believe that you can wipe out a percentage of the infection with each dose; but at the rate H. pylori replicate, I think other tools need to be used as well to take care of the whole problem. That's why people seem to see improvements when they use bee propolis or mastic gum, but the problem often multiplies again as soon as they discontinue use.

Since bee propolis and mastic gum also have the ability to wipe out good bacteria, using probiotics for a couple weeks after you are done using the bee propolis or mastic gum may be a good idea. It seems like people do well with two or three capsules of bee propolis or mastic gum twice a day on an empty stomach—first thing when waking up and again right before going to bed.

APPENDIX B

Intermediate Testing Procedures

Here I include procedures for intermediate tests that you can run yourself to acquire more information about yourself. You should have already read chapters five and six before jumping into these intermediate testing procedures.

To get the most from these intermediate testing procedures, you will need to include the results from your simple self-tests from chapter five. Be sure to have your filled-in *Data Tracking Sheet* handy so you can include that data along with any new findings from the intermediate tests discussed here. The simple tests from chapter five include:

- pH of Urine and Saliva
- Blood Pressure
- Breath Rate
- Breath Hold Time
- Blood Glucose

Many of the tests explained in this appendix will not only provide more information about the imbalances discussed in this book, they could also give insight to additional imbalances that were not covered in the main chapters. In Appendix C you will learn about the Sympathetic/Parasympathetic Imbalances, and the Acid/Alkaline Imbalances.

To perform one of these intermediate tests, you will need to get a pack of 11-parameter testing strips. You can find these urinalysis reagent test strips on Amazon.com. Some brands may sell only 10-parameter testing strips. These varieties will work just as well. Cybow is one of the brands I often use because they are very affordably priced at around $10-$15.

If you have acquired the tools needed to run the intermediate tests, go to www.KickItNaturally.com and click BOOK TOOLS to download an *Intermediate Imbalance Guide* to use for these procedures. You will input the information from these procedures onto the *Intermediate Imbalance Guide* instead of the basic version. You will learn how to fill out this guide later in this appendix.

These are great tests that everyone should run initially, if you have the ability to do so. You won't need to run most of these tests as often as the frequently used tests from chapter five, but they can still provide excellent information as you get started.

Resting to Standing - Blood Pressure Test

To get an indication of how your body is recovering from a given stress, you can perform a "resting to standing" blood pressure reading. You will actually take your blood pressure reading two times in a row during this test.

1. To test your resting blood pressure: Lie down and test on your left arm according to the directions for your blood pressure cuff, just like you did previously in your normal resting blood pressure test in chapter five.
2. To test your standing blood pressure: Remain in a lying position, push the button to start the inflation again, then stand up and hold your arm still as not to disturb the machine from taking its reading. You may need to have the machine in your other hand so you can hold it as still as possible as you get up. If the tube from the cuff to the machine is long enough, setting the machine on a table next to you is the best option. If the tube is not long enough, you will have to try to hold the machine as still as possible (along with holding yourself as still as possible) so the machine will not show an error code and require you to retest. If you do get an error code, you will want to lie back down for about 30 seconds to relax and do both steps one and two again.

Since you won't likely perform this test very often, a space is not reserved for it on the *Data Tracking Sheet*. Instead, just place both resting and standing readings on each line separated by a slash. For example, your systolic pressure line might look like this: 122/130. The 122 would indicate your systolic (top) number while you were lying down and the 130 would represent your systolic number when you were standing up. Then, you can do the same thing for your diastolic and pulse numbers. The ideal result is to see your standing systolic reading higher than your resting systolic reading. If the standing number is lower, this can be an indication that the system may be having a hard time recovering from a given stress.

Dermographic Line

To perform this test, run the non-ink side of a pen across the inside of your arm and then wait 20-30 seconds to see if your skin turns red, white, or the mark just disappears. If the mark disappears, you would be considered balanced in this test.

This is an autonomic nervous system indicator. Typically if a person's vascular system is constricted, the dermographic line stays with a white center and can indicate the individual is leaning too far on the sympathetic side. If the dermographic line stays red, that can indicate a person is leaning toward the parasympathetic side.

Gag Reflex

Gag reflex is another indicator of the autonomic nervous system. High gag reflex is indicating that a person is leaning toward the parasympathetic side. The lack of a gag reflex indicates a leaning toward the sympathetic side. No test is required here. Simply ask yourself, if I'm brushing my teeth and the toothbrush goes a little too far back, do I have a tendency to gag?

Pupil Size

Pupil size is another indicator of the autonomic nervous system. Small pupils indicate parasympathetic; large pupils indicate sympathetic. Looking at the colored area of your eye, if your pupils cover less than 25% of that space, they can be considered small. If your pupils cover more than 50% of the colored area, they can be considered large. If your pupils take up between 25% - 50% of the colored space, this can be considered normal.

11-Parameter Urine Dipstick

On the website, www.Amazon.com, you can search for a product, Cybow Urinalysis Test Strips. You will likely find 10-parameter and 11-parameter versions. Either of these products will work. A canister of 100-125 test strips will run you $10-$15 and very few people will need to order these more than once. (Again, I am not partial to this brand, but they are often the easiest to find on Amazon.) These urinalysis test strips (also referred to as a 10-parameter or 11-parameter urine test strip) measure blood, urobilinogen, bilirubin, protein, nitrite, ketones, ascorbic acid, glucose, pH, specific gravity and leukocytes, in urine. Not only can these measurements help you recognize which imbalances may be the most severe for you, but also these measurements could uncover some fairly major issues that could cause all kinds of trouble if undetected. In my opinion, with these test strips, people can uncover information that is very meaningful—all for about ten cents a strip.

When using an 11-parameter urine test strip, all of the measurements can be read right away except the leukocytes reading. You want to start a two-minute timer as soon as you dampen the test strip and read the leukocytes box right at that two minute time. Pee into a cup and then dip the strip all the way into the cup. You may have to bend the strip a little by pushing the strip against the bottom of the cup in order to get all the colored boxes covered in urine. Pull the strip out right away and touch its edge on a paper towel to wick away some of the excess urine. Read the colors against the color chart on the strips container. On the *Data Tracking Sheet*, circle the colored boxes that match the colors on your dipstick for each reading.

This dipstick is a great, cheap way to look at some more in-depth numbers. I recommend using this 11-parameter dipstick at least once to get a bigger picture of what is going on with your body. Of course, you'll want to perform repeat tests if the dipstick test indicates a problem that you need to track. As I explain each parameter, understand that some of the words are all big and fancy. I just want to let you know what's available on these dipsticks. In this section, I give you a quick blurb about some of these variables. I don't spend time defining what some of these terms mean. Instead, I just let you know what indications they can provide.

Non-Hemolyzed / Hemolyzed
Blood should not be seen in urine. If it is, that could be an indication of either kidney or bladder distress or trauma. Sometimes non-hemolyzed blood can be seen during a woman's monthly cycle; if that is the case, the test should be administered again at a different time of the month.

Bilirubin
Bilirubin should not be seen in the urine. When bilirubin is seen in the urine, that means it did not go out the biliary pathway, down through the intestines and out the south gate (your butt). It is a validator that the biliary pathway isn't running as nicely as it should. Since bile flow is so important for digestion and waste removal, this is an excellent parameter to have access to.

Urobilinogen
Urobilinogen is not normally seen in urine. Urobilinogen is bilirubin that has been eaten for lunch in the intestines by bacteria. When bacteria eats bilirubin, they poop urobilinogen. This can be common if an individual is constipated.

Protein
Protein should not be seen in the urine. If it is, that can be an indicator that the kidneys may be overwhelmed. Protein in the urine can also be an indicator that the body is breaking down its own tissue.

Nitrite
A positive reading for nitrite is one of the indicators of a UTI (urinary tract infection)—some type of bacteria in the bladder.

Ketones
Ketones are produced by the burning of fat. Typically diabetics show ketones because they are not burning carbohydrates, they are burning fat. People on the Atkins Diet were given ketone strips to show that they had reached the goal of ketosis, so that they would burn fat. I'm not saying this is your goal. This parameter can help indicate if your body is predisposed to burn more fat or more glucose.

Ascorbic Acid
Ascorbic acid will alter the readings on the dipstick. So while this reading lets you know how much ascorbic acid might be being excreted in the urine, it also alerts you that some of the reagents may react improperly when there is too much ascorbic acid.

Glucose
The dipstick color chart shows that some glucose in the urine is "normal." I might agree that is "common" however one would not want to conclude that it is optimal or "normal." I don't feel it is correct that glucose should be in people's urine. Typically you see a glucose reading in the negative box, showing no glucose—that is how you want to see it.

pH
I already talked about pH in chapter five. This is just nice to have on the strip so you can conveniently check pH with all the other parameters.

Specific Gravity
Specific gravity can be used to validate whether or not your body is leaning too anabolic or too catabolic. This alone is not an indication, however, it can be a great piece of data when looking for further confirmation.

Leukocytes
If you see both leukocytes and nitrite in the urine, that is a very positive indicator of a urinary tract infection and bacteria in the bladder.

Bonus Test - Hemochromatosis

Hemochromatosis is also known as iron overload. Women who still get their period regularly have a much lower risk of experiencing any iron overload conditions since you bleed out iron every month. All the same, since excessive iron levels can cause so much trouble, it's really smart to know your iron levels before you start to use any iron supplements. You can find out for free by donating blood. When you donate blood to the Red Cross, they will always check your iron levels first to make sure you can afford to give up any iron before they start draining blood out of your arm like a giant mosquito. If your iron is too low, they won't let you donate. They will prick your finger and put a drop of your blood into a little box that will output a number indicating your blood iron levels. Below 12.5, they won't let you donate. It is not likely that your number will exceed 15; but if it does, you may want to have a full iron panel done at a lab. I will provide you with a website where you can order one through the Internet, without a doctor's prescription, since it is used only for educational purposes.

There is a hereditary DNA malfunction, hemochromatosis, which is very common for men of Irish or Scottish descent. I am both Irish and Scottish, yet 23 doctors never figured out that I have hemochromatosis. Even though my iron levels were through the roof, nobody picked up on it. One doctor even asked me if I eat a lot of spinach. I told him no and he simply said, "Good, don't." That was it. Seeing that there is no reasonable drug or expensive procedure to correct hemochromatosis, it simply isn't in a doctor's ongoing education, since that education is most commonly provided by pharmaceutical companies.

Iron overload issues are not often a problem with constipation (although iron supplements do have the ability to lead to constipation). I simply want to add this information to all of our titles to spread awareness of this problem, especially for males (or females who no longer have a period) who are of Irish or Scottish descent. The medical world has removed the iron panel from most standard blood tests to cut down on costs, but they will add it on your test for free if you ask. You just have to know to ask. This condition is very easily treated if you know it is a problem for you. If you don't know, it can certainly cause a world of trouble and baffle doctor after doctor, run up a six figure medical bill, and flat out be annoying.

In the past, I have used the website www.healthcheckusa.com to order iron panels without a doctor's prescription. You simply buy the test online (it will run you about $60) and they email you a form to take into the lab. You just show up with the form and they draw a blood sample. You'll get your results back in a week or two. You may need a professional to help you interpret them, but the result sheet usually at least indicates if specific numbers are high or low. If your numbers are high, the same website also has a hemochromatosis DNA test you can order to find out if you carry any hemochromatosis genes.

It's all about education. There is now a wide variety of tests that you can order online in this manner. It's very easy to do and most tests are reasonably priced. It really works just like when your doctor sends you to a lab for a test, but in this scenario, the test results are sent to the online company and they send you a copy too (either by mail or email). There is value in consumers having the ability to learn about their own bodies so there are companies that can make this happen without a doctor.

Learn More

To learn more about advanced testing equipment or where you can take courses teaching how to use advanced testing methods, contact us at www.KickItNaturally.com. On this same site, you can also click on BOOK TOOLS > ADVANCED TESTING DETAILS, to read about more tests.

Sorting Out The Data

On the *Intermediate Imbalance Guide*, you see that some items have special symbols next to them. The items with a dagger symbol (†) are measurements that you use the 11-parameter urine dipsticks to acquire. The delta symbol (Δ) indicates measurements acquired with use of a special set of equipment or with help from a professional. You can see that you can gain quite a lot of info with just the basic tests that were outlined in chapter five, using tools like pH strips, a blood pressure cuff, and a stopwatch or egg timer.

You can follow along as I go through each measurement on the *Intermediate Imbalance Guide*. Many measurements are self-explanatory, but there are a few that I describe in a little more detail because they could use extra clarification. You can then use this as a reference tool as you're filling out your *Intermediate Imbalance Guide*. You don't want to check off an item if you don't really understand what it means. Having blank items is normal and should be expected. You want to check off only the items that are clearly a problem for you. For example, under catabolic, you see "Soft/Loose Stool." Check it off only if that is something you have been experiencing frequently, over the last month or so. Don't just check it off because you went to Mexico once and had some butt soup for two weeks. In that same regard, don't say you're not constipated if you're using two tablespoons of Milk of Magnesia every day in order to see any movement. Check off only the things that are apparent for you regularly so you don't sway your "snapshot" and make yourself look like someone you're not.

Imbalance Guide Content

Symbols Key

< less than (i.e. Pulse < 70 means Pulse is less than 70)
> greater than (i.e. Glucose > 100 means Glucose is greater than 100)
† requires an 11-parameter urine dipstick
Δ requires special equipment or a professional

Electrolyte Status

For both of the imbalances under "Electrolyte Status," the numbers are pretty self-explanatory. *Resting Systolic BP* is the top number of your blood pressure while you are lying down or resting in a seated position. *Standing Diastolic BP* is the bottom number of your blood pressure while you are in a standing position. *Pulse* is the number that comes up on the very bottom of most automatic blood pressure cuffs (for this form you want to use the pulse from the lying or seated position). Some individuals have a pulse that skips beats. These individuals should understand that this is unacceptable, even though it is often seen by professionals as "normal." It's best to regard a skipping pulse as far from "ideal." This issue can be time sensitive enough to talk to a health professional.

Imbalance - Electrolyte Deficiency

- Low Blood Pressure (Resting Systolic BP < 112)
- Standing Diastalolic BP < 73
- Pulse < 70

Imbalance - Electrolyte Excess

- High Blood Pressure (Resting Systolic BP > 130)
- Standing Diastolic BP > 87

Circadian Rhythm (Cellular Permeability)

Imbalance - Anabolic

- Urine pH > 6.3
- Saliva pH < 6.6
- † Specific Gravity < 1.011
- Low Debris in Urine (This means that if you have your urine in a clear cup, you really won't see much floating around in there. Anabolic people are usually stuck in the rebuilding state, so they're not doing a lot of breaking down of old tissues or cells and the amount of debris found in the urine is much lower. You see the opposite under the catabolic state as a catabolic individual seems to always be peeing out junk the body is throwing away.)
- Hard Stool/Constipation
- High Body Temp
- Polyuria (Polyuria means frequent urination.)
- Difficult to Rise (Meaning the snooze button might be your best friend.)
- Δ Adjusted Surface Tension > 69
- Δ Saliva mS < 4.5
- Δ Urine rH2 High

Imbalance - Catabolic

- Urine pH < 6.1
- Saliva pH > 6.9
- † Specific Gravity > 1.020
- Soft/Loose Stool
- Oliguria (Infrequent urination, or frequent but in small amounts.)
- † Protein on Dipstick (This can be a strong catabolic marker because it's an indication that the body is breaking down tissues in the body. The protein that you're seeing here is protein from bodily tissues and usually not protein from a chicken sandwich.)
- Wake Easily
- Low Body Temp
- High Debris in Urine
- Migraines (A true migraine starts in the back of the head or the neck. The word "migraine" has come to describe any really bad headache, but not all headaches are truly migraines. If your headaches start at the front or top of your head, don't check this item.)

- Δ Adjusted Surface Tension < 67
- Δ Saliva mS > 5.5
- Δ Urine rH2 Low

Energy Production

Imbalance - Carb Burner

- Breath Rate > 18bpm (The "bpm" stands for breaths per minute. Remember, each inhale counts as one. Don't count on both the inhale and the exhale.)
- Breath Hold < 45sec
- Low Blood Pressure (Resting Systolic BP < 112)
- Δ Glucose < 70 (I categorized this in the "need equipment" group, but you could do this test with a glucometer that can be picked up at any pharmacy.)
- Urine pH > 6.3
- Saliva pH < 6.6
- Irritable When Hungry

Imbalance - Fat Burner

- Breath Rate < 14bpm
- Breath Hold > 60sec
- High Blood Pressure (Resting Systolic BP > 133)
- Δ Glucose > 100
- Urine pH < 6.1
- Saliva pH > 6.9
- Type II Diabetes

Autonomic Nervous System

Imbalance - Parasympathetic

- Small Pupils
- Pulse Pressure < 37 (The pulse pressure is a measurement found by subtracting your Resting Diastolic BP number from your Resting Systolic BP number. This number is your pulse pressure. When you register on *The Coalition* and input your blood pressure numbers into the progress charts, the charts will automatically calculate your pulse pressure for you and display it on the graph as well.)

- Gag Reflex Increased (If you brush your teeth and your toothbrush goes a little further back, do you gag? When you go to the dentist, do you gag?)
- Red Dermographic Line (With this test, you run the non-ink, round end of a pen across the inside of your arm and then wait 20-30 seconds to see if your skin turns red, white, or the mark just disappears. If the mark disappears, you don't need to add a check here. If it turns white, you'll place the check under "White Dermographic Line" in the Sympathetic section.)
- Low Body Temp (Below 98.6 degrees Fahrenheit. It should probably be at least a full point below or above before you would check this box or the high body temp box under sympathetic.)
- Warm Dry Hands
- Fingertips Warmer than Triceps (This is too hard to test on yourself since your triceps are the back of your upper arm, but you can have someone grab your fingertips and your triceps at the same time and tell you which is warmer. I recommend not having someone on the subway help you with this. Awkward.)
- Allergies
- Asthma

Imbalance - Sympathetic

- Large Pupils
- Pulse Pressure > 46
- Gag Reflex Decreased (You generally don't have a gag reflex.)
- White Dermographic Line
- High Body Temp
- Cold Hands
- Fingertips Colder than Triceps

Acid/Alkaline Balance

Imbalance - Tending to Acidosis

- Breath Rate > 18bpm
- Breath Hold < 41sec
- Shortness of Breath

Imbalance - Tending to Alkalosis

- Breath Rate < 14bpm

- Breath Hold > 64sec

Digestive Issues

- Low Blood Pressure (Resting Systolic BP < 112)
- Standing Diastolic BP < 73
- Burping or Bloating (Many people don't really understand what bloating means. If you ask a woman, "Do your clothes fit tighter at night than when you put them on in the morning?" and she says, "Yes," she's bloating. As far as burping goes, I'm not talking about a huge belch. But if you have little burps after a meal, that is burping. Many people don't even notice that they burp until you ask them and they'll come back a day later and say, "Ya know, I really do burp.")
- Passing Gas
- Reflux/Heartburn
- Δ Total Ureas < 13
- Light Colored Stool (Either it is lighter than the color of corrugated cardboard, or your stool color will vary from light to dark depending on what you eat.)
- Constipation
- Urgent Diarrhea
- Nausea
- Δ rH2 > 20 or Δ rH2 < 17.5
- † Bilirubin on Dipstick

Okay, I Can Add Check Marks... Now What?

Once you've gone through the *Intermediate Imbalance Guide* and added a check mark next to each piece of information that applies to you, you're ready to begin getting to know yourself. As you look over each imbalance box, the idea is just to see if one side has more check marks than the other side, and by how much. An entire box could have almost no check marks, or the check marks could be evenly distributed to both sides. Either of those options can be an indication of balance in that area. However, if you have more check marks on one side of an imbalance box than you do on the other side, that can be an indication of an area that could use some work. You're going to have to use your judgment here. Having one check mark on one side, and none on the other side, is hardly evidence of an imbalance. I really like to see at least a 30% increase of the check marks on one side compared to the other side before I start to consider there to be any imbalance. Of course, in most cases, I usually consider measurements to be more influential than symptoms.

Don't confirm an imbalance with just symptoms. If you have a few symptoms that are common for an imbalance, but none of your numbers point in that direction, I don't usually view that as enough to point me in any one direction. I really want to let the chemistry guide me and then use symptoms as tools of confirmation that the chemistry is an accurate picture. If an imbalance appears to be strong, go to the bottom of the *Intermediate Imbalance Guide* and circle that imbalance. If it looks like you could be leaning that direction, but it's not so bad, you can just underline the imbalance to indicate that it needs work, but may not be your biggest trouble area. While evaluating your numbers, also look at how far out of range your numbers are. For example, if your systolic blood pressure is 89, that's a pretty long way from 112 so you can add more weight to that particular parameter. If your systolic blood pressure is 111, yes, that is still below range, but you may have just caught yourself at a low point and you'll want to test that number a couple more times over the next week or so. This allows you to see how you're trending. Obviously, how your numbers are trending over multiple measurements is a more complete picture than a single measurement. This is why the graphs on the Coalition are so useful. A person can begin to see improvements over a longer period of time. Healing is a slower, agricultural effort compared to symptom relief.

When you test all your numbers, you're really looking at a range. You don't know if the day that you tested is an example of your best day or your worst day. That is why you will continue to check the simple self-tests a couple times a week so you can start to look for patterns in your numbers. If your systolic blood pressure is below 95 every time you test it, you know it's low. Just keep in mind that you're not using NASA equipment. It's just a blood pressure cuff you picked up at the pharmacy, right next to where they sell condoms that are ribbed for her enjoyment. It's probably not high-tech stuff or it wouldn't be sold right next to the contraceptive devices. You may often notice that you can check your blood pressure and see a systolic of 101 and then check it a few minutes later and see a systolic of 92. That's okay. Those are both low and you at least understand the range that you are in. It is the same with pH strips. You're using pH strips that are just indicating a measurement that you're interpreting through a color, you're not using a pH meter that's accurate to the hundredth.

Conclusions

Once you've completed this process, make your conclusions just like you did in chapter six. The only difference is you now have more data to guide your decision-making process. In Appendix C you can read more details about all of the imbalances covered in this section.

APPENDIX C

Imbalances

I like to include an explanation of all ten imbalances in the appendix of all of my books. This allows you to use this section as a reference source and gives me the chance to cover any imbalances that may not be covered from book to book. With that in mind, some of this material may be review for you. However, since I didn't yet cover four of the imbalances in this book, I include explanations of the Sympathetic and Parasympathetic Imbalances, and the Acid and Alkaline Imbalances here.

Electrolyte State

The electrolyte state is defined by blood pressure (though a professional health coach may have equipment that can look at other variables in this equation, like conductivity of urine and saliva). In the world of natural health, where the terrain of the body gives so many insights into how the body is functioning, if an imbalance can exist in one direction, there must be an opposite to that imbalance. Otherwise, there would be no middle ground, no place where the body could be considered "balanced." Seems reasonable, right?

Imbalance - Electrolyte Deficiency

Very few doctors will ever complain about your blood pressure being low. Since there is no drug that is labeled for low blood pressure, the ramifications are not in their training. We all know that high blood pressure can cause heart attacks and strokes (blowouts). When they say your blood pressure is great even though it's too low, they're saying that you'll never have a blowout. But is it fun to run around on flat tires all day? An optimal blood pressure reading is said to be 120 over 80. So, if 140 over 90 is considered high blood pressure in the medical world, wouldn't having those numbers off by the same amount in the other direction be regarded as low blood pressure? Shouldn't a reading of 100 over 70 be considered low?

When blood pressure is low, this is often a reflection of low mineral content in the bloodstream. When the mineral levels decrease, it is a reflection of a decrease in your salts or the vascular system being too open (dilated). Our mineral content not only comes from actual salt, but from our food too. If your digestion is not working properly, you can't assimilate the minerals from the food you're eating and the mineral content in the system can decrease. (I go over this in more detail when I talk about digestion in chapter three.) There are a few other possible contributing factors that can result in low blood pressure. In most cases, however, digestion is the most prevalent contributing factor to low blood pressure. When we see low blood pressure, for example, anything lower than a systolic reading (the top number) of 112 and a diastolic reading (the bottom number) lower than 73, we consider that there is likely an Electrolyte Deficiency Imbalance present.

The minerals, or salts, in the system represent the conductivity, or ability for electricity to flow through the system. When the mineral content is low, there's no spark; and energy can be low. Without this energy, the brain can't function at its full potential, a result created by the lack of minerals required for signals to travel through. Many people with depression, and even other manifestations of "mental illness," are often just cases where there is not enough mineral in the system. Low mineral levels often mean there's not enough spark to give the brain what it needs to function correctly, or there is not enough mineral to control blood pH sufficiently.

Possible symptoms that can show up with an Electrolyte Deficiency Imbalance:
- chronic fatigue
- low blood pressure
- menstrual cramps
- poor circulation
- decreased libido
- depression or anxiety
- vertigo or dizziness when standing

- cravings
- insomnia

Imbalance - Electrolyte Excess

If an Electrolyte Deficiency Imbalance normally indicates a lack of electrolytes, the opposite would be a state where too many electrolytes are present. This is called an Electrolyte Excess Imbalance.

In general, high blood pressure can be an expression of insufficient, or lousy, kidney function. This means that, when excessive electrolytes become concentrated in the bodily fluids, it's usually a result of insufficient hydration (not drinking enough clean water) or impaired excretion of mineral salts through the kidneys. High blood pressure can also result from a constricted vascular system. In any case, electrolyte stress can lead to hypertension (high blood pressure) and other circulatory and cardiovascular problems. A vascular system that is constricted often points to an autonomic nervous system issue or a buildup on the arterial walls. (I talk more about the autonomic nervous system in the section about Sympathetic and Parasympathetic Imbalances later in this appendix.)

Stiffening arterial walls can lift pulse pressure, which is the difference between the systolic and diastolic blood pressure numbers. When the pulse pressure becomes greater and greater as the arterial walls become stiffer and stiffer, the heart becomes weaker and weaker. If you are a person with high blood pressure who is trying to bring it down naturally, watching the pulse pressure correct itself helps to validate that you are doing the right thing. Remember, *The Coalition for Health Education* has a tool that calculates your pulse pressure for you so you can just monitor the changes without worrying about the math or really understanding what pulse pressure is.

Possible symptoms that can show up with an Electrolyte Excess Imbalance:
- high blood pressure
- hardening of the arteries
- heart attack
- stroke
- poor circulation
- inability to properly transport oxygen, nutrients, waste products, antibodies and more, throughout your system

Catabolic/Anabolic States

At the cellular level, the body is always in an anabolic or catabolic state, or in the process of switching back and forth between the two. During the day, our cell membranes are intended to open up (much like a flower) so nutrients can get in and out more easily. This "more open" state is called a catabolic state. At night, our cell membranes are intended to become more closed (again, like a flower) so nutrients cannot get in and out as easily. This "more closed" state is called an anabolic state. Cells don't actually open and close like a flower, this is just a "basic" view that allows us to talk about the different states of our cells. Both states are appropriate, and even necessary, for a body to function optimally. Due to many possible factors, some people can get stuck in one state and their body will not switch back and forth as intended.

To make the body operate correctly, we need to oscillate back and forth from the anabolic state at night, while we sleep, and a catabolic state during the day, while we're active. Without this natural oscillation, many problems can occur. When the body shifts from anabolic to catabolic, that's when the endorphins in the brain are released, which can help people from becoming depressed. Though there are many other factors that more commonly contribute to depression, you see that this natural oscillation between the anabolic and catabolic states can be important.

Imbalance - Anabolic

First of all, there are many benefits that take place while a body is in an anabolic state. This is the state where the body engages in most of its repairing or rebuilding processes. You've probably heard the word anabolic in reference to steroids. Weightlifters take anabolic steroids in order to be in the tissue building, anabolic state when they are not playing fair with muscle building.

While an anabolic state can have its benefits, any state can cause problems when pushed to an extreme. Although it is very appropriate for the cells to be in an anabolic state at night, some individuals will stay in a more anabolic state most of the time. These individuals are said to be experiencing an Anabolic Imbalance.

If you're stuck in an anabolic state most of the time, it can be very hard to get up in the morning because your body, at the cellular level, is actually still in sleep mode. In the same way that many people who suffer from insomnia are stuck in a catabolic state where their body is always awake, anabolic people can have a hard time getting their bodies in motion in the morning. The snooze button can be their best friend. Be sure to understand, however, that everyone who experiences insomnia is not necessarily stuck in a catabolic state. There are aspects to an Anabolic Imbalance that can also cause insomnia for totally different reasons. You can learn more about insomnia by going to www.KickItNaturally.com and searching for our insomnia podcast episode. Please don't think that, if you suffer from insomnia, you must not have an Anabolic Imbalance because a Catabolic Imbalance is only one possible cause for insomnia. There are insomnia cases that exist quite well in an anabolic state too. Also, don't think that if you pop right out of bed in the morning that you can't have an Anabolic Imbalance. Remember, imbalances can show their heads in different ways for different people. There are no "rules" to follow, only guidelines to help you along.

This Anabolic Imbalance can also cause constipation by sending too much of the body's water to the kidneys and not enough to the bowels, making the stool harder and more difficult to move. An Anabolic Imbalance can also cause individuals to pee high volumes of urine frequently throughout the day. They will often have to get up in the middle of the night to tinkle.

Possible symptoms that can show up with an Anabolic Imbalance:
- constipation or hard stool
- tachycardia (rapid heart rate)
- anxiety/panic attacks
- frequent urination
- difficulty waking in the morning
- viral problems

Be sure not to just assume you have an imbalance because you're experiencing some (or even all) of the symptoms that commonly show up with that imbalance. Without looking at your specific chemistry, and understanding how your body is operating, and what is causing your issues, you're really just throwing darts when you try to treat symptoms that way.

Imbalance - Catabolic

When it comes to cellular permeability, the catabolic state is the opposite of the anabolic state. It's the other side of the coin. The catabolic state is where the body kind of "breaks down and cleans house," so to speak. In a catabolic state, the body is primed to use oxygen to create energy, so it is appropriate to be in a catabolic state during your waking hours to keep you going all day. This, along with what I just explained about the anabolic state, helps to show how both the anabolic and catabolic states are appropriate during the appropriate (day and night) times. However, in the same way that I talked about people who lean too anabolic, some individuals will stay in a more catabolic state most of the time. These individuals are said to be experiencing a Catabolic Imbalance.

If someone is stuck in a catabolic state, the cell walls are too permeable and this individual will often burn up muscle and protein and even membrane fats. Breaking down tissues and muscle so they can be rebuilt is a beneficial aspect of the catabolic state, but when a person is in that state too often, for too long, that "cleaning house" process can turn into a body that is flat out falling apart. The more muscle we lose, the lower our metabolism, and we may burn less fat.

Insomnia is very common with a Catabolic Imbalance because the cell membranes appear to be more permeable, which is a characteristic of the daytime state. These people can't sleep because their bodies are still awake and operating at full speed. Most sleeping aids will knock you out in the head so you can sleep, but your body will still be wide awake all night. As a result, you might either wake up exhausted or you become tired again a few hours after waking.

Possible symptoms that can show up with a Catabolic Imbalance:
- insomnia
- migraines
- chronic diarrhea or loose stool
- hair falling out
- muscle loss
- chronic pain
- loss of connective tissue or difficulty in healing

- aging quickly
- joint and muscle pain; arthritis (especially rheumatoid)
- oliguria (insufficient urination, perhaps often but in small amounts)
- low body temperature
- bacterial problems

Since an overly catabolic state is sometimes described as a lack of sterols at the cellular level, increasing your intake of sterols and saturated fatty acids, such as real butter or coconut oil, can be one method to help improve this imbalance. However, I find that most individuals with this imbalance also need to use more nutrients like specific vitamins, minerals and amino acids in order to see lasting improvement. That being said, increasing your sterol intake while optimizing digestion can be a great place to start.

Energy Production

The next two imbalances I cover are Fat Burner Imbalance and Carb Burner Imbalance. These deal with energy production and how the body uses food for fuel. Before I explain energy production, understand that I will be leaving out complicated methods the body can use to create energy. They are not important for this explanation.

To create energy, simply speaking, our bodies burn either fat or glucose. Your body is designed to burn both types of fuel for different purposes. Despite that, changes can occur in our bodies, or in our lives, that will train our bodies to prefer one fuel over the other. The body may stop burning the other type of fuel almost entirely. This is another reason why there is no such thing as the diet that is right for everyone. It doesn't exist. Some people burn fats much better than glucose and some people are the opposite. This really puts all these arguments into perspective about "low-carb," "low-fat," "high-protein," "the drunk diet," "I only eat things that start with the letter F..." I could go on for days. They're still all going to be wrong for most folks. In order to find the right "diet," you really need to look at a person's digestive capacity and their biological individuality, because each person processes foods differently.

Imbalance - Carb Burner

Carb Burners are people who are predisposed to burn off all their glucose and do not seem to burn fat very well. Now, it's not that they won't burn fat, but they will always prefer to burn off all their glucose first. This is commonly referred to as hypoglycemia. Just keep in mind that the hypoglycemic can also be a step away from becoming diabetic. "But if he's hypoglycemic, how can he be a step away from becoming diabetic?" It's because many hypoglycemics have way too much insulin in the system and their system responds as though there are five furnaces in the house. Every time the house gets cold, instead of one furnace coming on and slowly warming up the house and then turning off, FIVE furnaces turn on and the house is hot enough to make you cuss by the time the furnaces shut down.

A Carb Burner's insulin can work in this same manner. These individuals have become insulin resistant, but they have not been insulin resistant long enough that the cells have stopped responding to the insulin altogether. They're at that stage where the cells are still responsive enough to the insulin that, when the pancreas produces up to five times the amount of insulin it normally would, it reaches a critical level and all the sugar goes into the cells at one time. These people can get very severe headaches in the front of their heads. They may also complain that their head feels full or they'll get fuzzy brained; this is due to the blood sugar dropping far too rapidly. Using a blood sugar glucometer can quantify that the blood glucose has gone too low. This low blood sugar can make these folks extremely miserable, and being around them when blood sugar levels drop can be equally miserable. If you live with, or if you are this person, you know exactly what I'm talking about.

Possible symptoms that can show up with a Carb Burner Imbalance:
- lack of energy; physical and mental fatigue
- high or low blood sugar
- shortness of breath
- high cholesterol
- overweight or underweight
- irritable when hungry

Imbalance - Fat Burner

If you find that you show indications of having a Fat Burner Imbalance, you most likely are burning much more fat than glucose. If you also have high cholesterol, high triglycerides and a high fasting glucose, any of these markers can be another indication that you are not processing glucose effectively.

Many individuals who are overweight and have this imbalance will ask, "How is it that I'm burning mostly fat but I'm still so fat?" This is because their bodies are turning almost every carb and sugar that they eat into fat. In order to process sugar or glucose, the body is having to take all sugar or glucose coming in and turn it into fat before it is able to be "burned" for energy.

Possible symptoms that can show up with a Fat Burner Imbalance:
- lack of energy; physical and mental fatigue
- Type II Diabetes
- metabolic syndrome (or insulin resistance)
- high blood pressure or cardiovascular disease
- weight gain
- gallbladder trouble
- high triglycerides

You may have noticed Type II Diabetes on the list above. This doesn't mean that if you have a Fat Burner Imbalance that you're diabetic. It just means that in this fat burning state, the body prefers to burn fat and can often move into a predicament where it will burn very little glucose, if any. In these cases, glucose can accumulate in the bloodstream and, abracadabra, you're insulin resistant and type II diabetic. Remember, I am only describing an imbalance in this section and not a disease. However, a neglected imbalance certainly can manifest itself eventually as a disease, just like neglecting to change the oil in your engine can manifest itself as a blown up engine.

By improving this imbalance and allowing the body to once again process both types of fuel, a person could increase energy and lose some weight, since such a large percentage of glucose would no longer need to be stored as fat.

Autonomic Nervous System

Sympathetic Dominance refers to the autonomic nervous system (ANS). The ANS is a mechanism in the body that happens without having to consciously think about it. You don't have to think about whether your heart is beating, it just does. The other side of the nervous system is the Parasympathetic Dominance.

The sympathetic side is the speed side—the fight-or-flight response. The parasympathetic side is the slow side—the rest-and-digest state. These two systems are hard-wired, in a sense, to the heart, the entire digestive system, and all the lower level glands, organs and systems.

Imbalance - Parasympathetic

A Parasympathetic Imbalance is often where I find individuals who suffer from allergies or asthma. This can be a tricky imbalance because if an individual has a strong ANS imbalance, especially on the parasympathetic side, that person can often see a response that is opposite of what is expected when working to balance the body. For example, if a specific food or supplement tends to push one measurement, like urine pH, down for most people, that same food or supplement could actually push up that measurement for a parasympathetic dominated person. I've never heard a good explanation as to why this can occur for some, but it seems the defense system and immunological issues affect this anomaly. It is seen frequently enough in parasympathetics that you need to know this anomaly exists. That is why learning to monitor your body is so important. Monitoring your body will also alert you when the time has come to get the help of a professional who understands the wide variety of nuances that can occur when looking at layer upon layer of imbalances and their priorities in the body.

Possible symptoms that can show up with a Parasympathetic Imbalance:
- allergies
- asthma
- small pupil size
- frequent urination
- increased saliva
- muscle cramps at night
- eyes or nose watery

- eyelids swollen
- gag easily
- poor circulation

Imbalance - Sympathetic

The ANS is reactive. As a stress situation presents itself, the system turns on, does its job, and in doing so possibly reaches its outer bounds of homeostasis (perfect balanced health). Thanks to this selfish act of the ANS, other systems in the body can be deprived and suffer. Not unlike the transmission in your car, systems in the body can "lock up" and refuse to shift out of low gear, thus causing a myriad of symptoms such as unpredictable and/or uncalled-for behavior. The stress situations that are instigating the reaction of the ANS could be emotional, nutritional, or mineral in origin. If individuals are stuck in a sympathetic state, they can feel stressed and on edge, and even have trouble sleeping since they are stuck in fight-or-flight mode.

Possible symptoms that can show up with a Sympathetic Imbalance:
- large pupil size
- low levels of urination
- increased temperature
- sweaty hands
- dry mouth/eyes/nose
- get chills often
- cold extremities (like hands or feet)
- unable to relax
- irritated by strong light

pH Balance - Acid/Alkaline Imbalances

Everybody just calm down. This can be a very hot topic in the world of natural health. If this book is your first taste of natural health, this section may open your eyes to some incredible things. Kind of like the series *LOST*, but this will actually make sense. However, if you have already read, or have been introduced to, information about the pH of the body, I may need to spend time fixing the damage that some other numskulls have created.

The bloodstream has a very narrow pH value that it must stay within in order for our bodies to function properly. If the blood moves too far acid or too far alkaline, we can literally die. The body doesn't want this to happen, so it does whatever it can to keep the bloodstream at a balanced pH level.

In the natural world, when people talk about pH, they frequently talk about how we all need to "alkalize." "Alkalize, alkalize, alkalize." "Alkalize or die a slow, miserable death," they tell us. These pH "gurus" explain how we are all too "acid" and it's killing us one by one. Of course, when someone follows these approaches and tries to alkalize themselves, and they completely fall apart, the guru tells them, "That's okay, you're going through a 'healing crisis'. Just stick to it and you'll be fine." No, what we're going through is a guru crisis. There currently appears to be a crisis where a few gurus need to be punched in the neck so maybe they will stop ruining the well-being of half of their readership.

These readers who started to fall apart after "alkalizing" themselves were likely falling apart because they were pushing an imbalance that already existed even further over the edge. Remember how I talked about the fact that an imbalance can't exist unless there is an equal imbalance in the other direction? If someone told you one pair of glasses will fix everyone's vision, you would question his intelligence or just poke him in the eye. We all know that reading glasses can help farsighted people while nearsighted individuals need the very opposite type of lens. Any author who tells the reader that EVERYONE should do ANYTHING is trying to sell something.

The haphazard confusion starts here: Some individuals truly are too "acidic." I talk about what this means in just a moment. For now, I'm going to continue using the same ignorant terminology that most of the pH gurus use. When individuals have an Acid Imbalance, and they truly can benefit from "alkalizing" themselves, these individuals can follow the instructions laid out by a pH guru and they may see tremendous improvement to their health, or at least their well-being. In some cases, these results could even be considered miraculous. Still, let's just calm down for a minute. If we know that every imbalance (like an Acid Imbalance) will have an opposite imbalance in the other direction, what are these pH gurus doing to the people who have an Alkaline Imbalance (the opposite of an Acid Imbalance)? They're making these individuals miserable and calling it a "healing crisis." That's what they're doing.

To go right along with all of the pH and alkalizing books and experts out there, we also find shelves upon shelves of "alkalizing" products in every health food store. You can't throw a stick down the aisle of a health food store without hitting a product that boasts its ability to improve your health through alkalizing. (By the way, if you do this, the employees will come right up to you and ask you not to throw sticks in their store anymore... like I'm the one doing something wrong here.) It is also likely that these products will increase in popularity since many people will reap benefits from their use. Many people with an acidity issue, that is. To understand the tragedy in this, let's go over the Acid and Alkaline Imbalances.

The most important thing to understand is this: When I discuss an Acid or Alkaline Imbalance in this series of books, I am talking about blood pH. Measuring urine pH and saliva pH in a context of breath rate and breath hold can be incredibly insightful and useful, but urine pH or saliva pH are not always an indication of the pH of the blood, as many pH gurus will have you believe. It's a nice story, it just happens to be a fictional one. I already showed you how to measure urine pH and saliva pH. For now, I'm just going to dig into blood pH since this is the crucial parameter when looking at an Acid or Alkaline Imbalance.

Imbalance - Tending to Alkalosis

Alkalosis is an imbalance where the bloodstream is too alkaline. When the blood leans alkaline, oxygen can't leave the bloodstream and go to the tissue level where it needs to be to help your body create the energy required to run properly. In science, this is known as the Bohr Effect.

If a doctor checked your oxygen levels, he would put a device called a pulse oximeter on you and he might tell you that your oxygen is great... you have plenty. But, if the bloodstream is too alkaline, the oxygen cannot be released from the bloodstream and go into the tissues where it can be used. The result: You can feel wiped out. The oxygen is there, it just can't get to the right location in order to be properly utilized. In an effort to correct this, when the bloodstream is too alkaline, the body will slow the rate at which you breathe. Carbon dioxide (CO_2) is acid inducing to the bloodstream so the body tries to reduce the amount that you breathe in order to hold on to more CO_2, allowing it to acidify the bloodstream. Pretty neat trick Mother Nature came up with, don't you think? By using the CO2 to acidify a bloodstream that is too alkaline, some oxygen can be released from the bloodstream and can make it to the tissue level.

Possible symptoms that can show up with an Alkaline Imbalance:
- chronic fatigue
- sleep apnea
- joint and muscle pain; arthritis
- allergies; asthma
- muscle cramps
- fluid retention

In regard to sleep apnea, many cases are caused by structural issues (such as a flap that doesn't seem to be flapping correctly), but almost as many are caused by a bloodstream that is too alkaline. The breath rate drops so low due to an overly alkaline bloodstream that eventually the body says, "I'm gonna acidify this bloodstream and get some oxygen down to the tissues where it needs to be even if it kills this guy," and this would show itself as sleep apnea symptoms.

By looking at all the trouble an overly alkaline bloodstream can cause, do you see how important it is to look at people as individuals and measure where they are before you start blabbing about how everyone needs to alkalize? Just because something brings about an amazing result for one person, doesn't mean that it's not going to turn someone else into a zombie. This is another example of how people are different. Why is that so hard for many people to grasp? I've met individuals who can't get enough Maury Povich; yet if you forced me to watch that show, I might not ever talk to you again. We know people are different in their preferences; if they weren't, how would John Tesh have a fan base at all? Since people can have different tastes, doesn't it make sense that they could have different chemistry as well?

Imbalance - Tending to Acidosis

The physiology in a person with Acidosis problems expresses too much acid (or H+) in the bloodstream. One cause can be an imbalance in potassium, or an inability of the kidneys to properly excrete the acid—and balance is lost. The breath rate in these individuals becomes accelerated because the kidneys, being unable to easily control the acid level in the bloodstream, can be helped by the lungs huffing off CO2, because CO2 acidifies the bloodstream. These individuals will normally have a short breath-holding time and a rapid breathing rate, exposing the fact that the kidneys are not having an easy time controlling the pH of the blood. This can be remedied (depending on the cause) by assisting the system to buffer the acids more effectively and excreting them. But this is not just a failure to excrete acids, it's a failure to buffer them. This helps us to understand why using foods or supplements in an effort to "alkalize" an individual can be so beneficial. This is how a pH guru can hit home runs with some people who will then think he is so brilliant. These people with the overly acid issues can really benefit by increasing the nutrients that can be used to buffer these acids. Even a broken clock is right twice a day.

An inability to properly digest protein can often be an issue in these cases since the biggest buffer of acids in the body is protein. Obviously, it is more profitable for the industry to sell green drinks and alkalizing supplements than it is to help people better digest their protein. Yet, in some cases, simply improving protein digestion can be a great step toward giving the body the tools it needs to buffer those acids on its own.

Possible symptoms that can show up with an Acid Imbalance:
- shortness of breath
- rapid heart rate
- poor retention of important mineral nutrients
- fluid retention
- poor function of your kidneys, lungs, adrenal glands and many other organs and glands
- digestive issues

Alkalizing Water And Water Filters

The first step in digging through this dung is to remember that some individuals have an Acid Imbalance. Their blood is tending toward being too acid. If this is you, one of these alkalizing water filters could certainly help you feel better if it was pushing your blood to a more balanced state. You would know if it was working or not if your breath rate started to come down. In this scenario, you would start to feel better and would tell all of your friends it was because of the "magic water" that was coming out of your water filter and you're so excited because you only have sixty-three more monthly payments before it is paid off.

Let's not stop there. To a lot of my clients, I will hold up a bottle and say, "Have you heard of this? It's called WATER!" because it's so obvious that they're not drinking any. Water is one of the most important components to our health and yet so few people drink enough to help their bodies wash out all the junk. They think that if they're drinking a soda or coffee, that's enough. "It has water in it," they tell me. But soda and coffee, or even sport drinks, are hardly a replacement for water. None of those beverages have the ability to truly hydrate the cells like water can. Most of those drinks just introduce more junk into the body rather than giving your body what it needs to wash junk out. But tell me this: If a guy pays $3000 for a water filter, do you think he might drink some water? You bet he will! He'll probably go fill up a glass every time he opens his checkbook or checks his bank statement. "Where the hell did all my money go? Oh yeah, I guess I should go get a glass of water."

When you take a person who hasn't been drinking any water, and you start getting H2O down his gullet, that can often be enough to turn his whole world around. You start to hydrate the body, you start to clear out junk. Pounds get dropped, joints become more flexible, all sorts of happy stuff can happen—just by adding some water. Too bad he could have done the same thing with a ninety-nine cent jug of spring water.

I'll call this water filter-mortgaging consumer "Bill." Bill tells his friend Tanya about this filter and talks her into buying too. (Certainly this is just about her health and has nothing to do with the fact that Bill will be making money off of Tanya's purchase.) But Tanya starts to feel worse. She's exhausted and finds it easier to just sit on the couch all day. If you checked Tanya's breath rate you might see that it's around eight. With a breath rate that low, it could be that Tanya's blood is leaning too alkaline and this alkalizing water is pushing that imbalance further into the abyss.

Since Tanya hears testimonial after testimonial from people who have improved their health by drinking this water, she thinks it must be something else that is bringing her down. It can't be the water because every multilevel marketing meeting she goes to plays loud music and people dance around because they feel so good. Meanwhile, Tanya's blood is so alkaline that oxygen can't get down to the tissues and she just wants to lay down on the floor until they turn off the Macarena.

When deciding if alkalizing water is right for you, it's crucial to look at breath rate and understand if your blood could benefit from drinking this water or if it's just going to make you worse. Even if you do have an Acid Imbalance, and drinking alkaline water could benefit you, be sure to continue to check your breath rate for improvement. You don't want to correct an Acid Imbalance so well that you create an Alkaline Imbalance. Monitoring yourself and your numbers is what this type of health movement is all about. It's not about finding something that makes you feel better and using that product until you die. It's about using something until your body is balanced and then reducing it until you don't need it anymore.

As a side note, remember that the first thing that water hits is your stomach. If you're drinking alkaline water with your food, that alkalinity is going to reduce the effectiveness of stomach acid levels that may already be too low.

APPENDIX D

Those Who Paved the Way

Dr. Carey Reams

Dr. Carey Reams was an agrarian. He did soil chemistry and he learned, primarily, how to make things grow in the soil. By people coming to him for help, he was pushed into biology and working with animals and humans. What remained at the root of his mentality was all this knowledge about what made produce grow exceptionally well. What needed to be done in order to bring the proper level of minerals into the produce? What got a result in the crop? There are a lot of stories about how Reams adjusted minerals in the soil to affect the growth of produce. If you wanted to do something in soil, he knew how to do it. That mentality was then brought forward into looking at health from a simple ground-up standpoint. Reams looked at the mineral content in a person, much like he looked at the mineral content in the soil.

Dr. Emanuel Revici

Dr. Emanuel Revici was all about looking at the cell's oil-based membrane and the proteins that are mixed in with it. He explained what was going on with the permeability of the cells. Through learning about cellular permeability, we came to understand that there is a natural tide to life, or a rhythm. This is where the anabolic/catabolic language comes into use. We see that during the daytime it is proper for a person to be in a catabolic state—when he is giving his energy to the day. Conversely, as surely as night falls and the dandelion flower closes, the anabolic state is entered and the person goes to sleep to rebuild and restore himself. Everyone needs to be cycling between these two states. As people lose their vitality or resilience, this tide of life becomes impeded and an individual can get stuck in the anabolic or catabolic state 24 hours a day. Without the necessary vitality to allow the natural oscillation process to continue, it is statistically true that those who become stuck in an anabolic state are more prone to viral issues occurring in their system. Those who have lost their resilience and are stuck in a catabolic state are more prone to bacterial issues. Now comes the reasonableness of the system where if a person is really oscillating every evening from catabolic to anabolic, and every morning from anabolic going back to catabolic, then the viruses don't have a home and the bacteria don't have a home because the system is oscillating. There is never a time when, for many days, there is a hospitable environment for those issues to take hold.

There is a good book about Dr. Revici, written by William Kelley Eidem, called *The Doctor Who Cures Cancer*. This is a story of Revici's life and work and is an excellent introduction into the intellect he provided us.

Thomas Riddick

Thomas Riddick understood colloidal suspensions. What is the bloodstream? It is a colloidal suspension. This is information that painters understand perfectly because, if you can't keep pigment in suspension, then it is going to separate, fall to the bottom of the can and harden. If that pigment falls out of suspension then you aren't going to sell much paint. You aren't going to get the pigment to the wall, it's not going to dry correctly and it isn't going to work. With Riddick's research, we came to understand a lot more about the heart and how to make the bloodstream flow easier so that the heart does not work so hard.

Certainly, when half of America is dying from a heart-related problem, we would be curious to know what to do to make things easier for the heart. That used to be understood before profit-driven thinking took over. I don't want that to sound like I'm bitter, I'm not. I do wish that those who put profit over the public's well-being could be locked in a room and forced to listen to old Menudo albums until they promise to change their ways, but I'm not bitter. I don't want you to think that I'm the type of person who would Menudo-style waterboard someone. Still, wouldn't the world be a better place? If this was taken care of, the only issues we would need to get rid of are smoking in public, people who stink, and those who drive slow in the left lane. Order restored.

Dr. Melvin Page

Dr. Melvin Page was a medical doctor whose research showed that proper nutritional balance in the body could not only improve the health of someone's teeth, but also the health of the body would coincide with the improvement of their dental health. He found that, when the calcium-to-phosphorus ratio was in a balanced proportion, the patient would present no cavities. (The actual proportion is ten-to-four in the blood, for those who like it when I say things that make me sound fancy. For those who say, "What the hell is he talking about?" just use the word "balanced.") Moving outside of this ratio would not only present cavities, but other health issues as well.

Dr. Page was also very interested in, and had a lot of success with, hormones. He found that you couldn't even get a good read on hormones if the blood sugar was elevated. For this reason, he would require avoidance of carbohydrates for at least 72 hours before any hormone testing was done. When we look around us today, with the rate that the population is having trouble with diabetes, hypoglycemia, and blood sugar issues, is it any wonder that there are also a lot of hormonal issues going on? Dr. Page had a lot of information that we try to implement.

Dr. Page and all these other doctors serve to validate or challenge each other's views. It's as though they're all looking into the same room (human physiology) but through different windows, giving a different perspective on very similar issues.

Recommended Reading

The Doctor Who Cures Cancer - William Kelley Eidem
> The story of Emanuel Revici, M.D. that introduced us to the anabolic/catabolic shifts in the body.

Nutrition and Your Mind - George Watson
> An excellent book that demonstrates how the types of foods we eat can make a difference in our physical health and mental health.

APPENDIX E

A Healthy Body In An Unhealthy World

Nobody can avoid everything that is bad for the human body. It's just not possible in the world we live in. Even if you cancel your DirecTV subscription, fire your dog walker, and move out into the woods, you can still have a bird fly over and poop in your mouth while you're sunbathing next to a natural stream. The trick is not to try to eliminate every toxin, chemical and pollutant from entering your body; but, instead, to put your body in a position where it can have an easier time of removing those problems. That's the whole point in improving the "flow" of the body and balancing the systems that make it all work.

While you're helping your body perform at a higher level, the next goal is merely to learn about the facets of your life that are contributing to your body's toxic load, then get rid of the ones that are the easiest for you to eliminate. Don't feel like you need to run in horror from every environmental or household pollutant within a thirty-mile radius or you're going to be doing some Forrest Gump-type running. However, if there are factors in your life that are easy for you to change, go ahead and change them. That will be one less irritant that your body has to deal with—one less task that it needs to take care of before it can move on to more important bodily processes.

It's my view that the body is more than capable of handling some of this junk. Worrying about every possible toxin is just going to create more stress, more harmful chemicals that accompany that stress, and more work for your body to do. Criminy Pete! Chill out and enjoy your life.

In this section, I also talk about items that many people feel are healthy solutions. I explain why these people are idiots. They may not truly be idiots—they may just be misled—but I'm going to call them idiots anyway, just because it's faster and easier. Bear in mind that almost every product, method or idea out there could benefit *somebody*. I think there are very few ideas that are completely invalid for the entire population. I just get annoyed when people try to push their products on everyone and market their products as if they are the solution to every human ailment existing today. I feel strongly that there is no such product; a lot of it has to do with what happens to be popular at any given moment. I mean, now it seems popular to watch shows about people getting screamed at in a kitchen. Who saw that coming?

Chemicals In Tap Water

I was at my brother's house in Florida this summer when we decided to use his pool testing kit to look at his tap water. We tested both his pool and the water from the tap in his kitchen. We both sort of freaked when we saw that there was more chlorine in his tap water than in his pool! What the...?! My brother freaked because he thought, "Man, I must really need more chlorine in my pool," and ran out to his shed to add more. But his pool wasn't green with algae; and it became clear the next day, as all of our eyes were burning in the pool during a game of paddle ball, that he really didn't need more chlorine in his pool—he needed less in his tap water.

Most city water treatment plants use both chlorine and fluoride to treat the water. Both of these chemicals are harmful to the human body in their own right. An immediate impact these chemicals can have on the body is their ability to "displace" iodine from the body. I say "displace" because that is how most researchers view what chlorine and fluoride are doing to iodine levels in the body. Though iodine levels do normally go down if consuming chlorine- and fluoride-laden water, I view this another way: Iodine acts as a disperser in the body. It disperses toxins so they can be removed from the system. The body views chlorine and fluoride as toxins. (Yes, I know your dentist told you fluoride was good for your teeth, but what he didn't tell you is that it is not good for your body... oops. He will also tell you mercury in your mouth isn't dangerous.) Therefore, iodine is used to help disperse these toxins. In essence, these chemicals are stripping, or displacing, the iodine from the system; but it makes more sense to view this as the body is using up its iodine to deal with this problem. In any event, an iodine deficiency can be created.

It is widely accepted that iodine is required for proper thyroid function, and thyroid "conditions" have been on the rise in the past decade or so. Although I feel that the rise of this epidemic has more to do with the rise in popularity of prescribing thyroid medications, it could also be partially due to the fact that cities are using more and more chemicals to treat our water. It is also important to consider that iodine is a mineral that can be difficult for some people to absorb. Some minerals are easier to absorb than others and come into the system even if the system is imbalanced. Iodine, on the other hand, requires a more balanced system in order to be absorbed properly. That's why giving iodine to patients with thyroid issues will often bring no result. You can dump all the iodine you want into a person; but if that iodine can't be absorbed, it's not going to help. This is why the medical world has shifted to using drugs in most thyroid cases.

The significance of this, in reference to water, is understanding that if people already have a low level of iodine, you can see how drinking tap water filled with chlorine or fluoride could really do a number on their iodine levels. Crazy to see how just drinking tap water could result in a thyroid issue, right? Yet, understanding the science makes it hard to argue.

Most filter pitchers filter the water through carbon which does very little to remove chlorine and fluoride from your tap water. When it comes to filters, I like the good reverse osmosis filters that can be installed under your sink; but even these filters can remove good minerals while they're removing the bad stuff. If you use a reverse osmosis filter, it's a good idea to add mineral drops back into your water. The company, Trace Minerals Research, makes a product called Concentrace Trace Mineral Drops. It's sold at most health food stores. Adding just three or four drops per glass of water can replenish minerals that may have been stripped during the filtration process. Of course, if you have high blood pressure, you would cut that dosage in half. Don't think these drops are going to give your body all the minerals that it needs. The best move is to improve digestion so you can pull more minerals out of your food. However, adding minerals to water that has been stripped of many of its minerals can have its benefits for some people.

Spring water is the best option, but it can be costly to buy. I don't really like the idea of distilled water for most people because it is void of any mineral whatsoever, and can wash away more mineral than spring water might. For some people, merely getting any form of water into them is going to be beneficial; so again, I don't want to split hairs with water for some. But since I'm talking about ways to reduce the intake of toxic substances, the type of water can be important.

Shower Filters

Now that you understand the trouble that chlorine can cause, let's hit the showers because most of us don't think about how the water we bathe in can affect our bodies. It's true that most of us don't drink the water coming out of the showerhead while we're washing our hair, but we do continue to breathe while we're showering. When that hot water turns into mist and steam, it still contains all the chemicals that are in that water. As we breathe in this steam, those chemicals come into our lungs then into our bloodstream even faster than if we were drinking the water. In a way, this could make the need to filter our shower water even more important than filtering the water we're drinking. Since this water has a faster path to your bloodstream, doing something to remove or reduce this chlorine can be a good idea.

This is a pretty easy fix and I have had a lot of people tell me they started feeling better after they added a shower filter. I myself was getting extremely tired after my showers and the only thought I could come up with was, "How long was I in there?!" I never considered that the steam in my shower was filling my lungs with chemicals that my body was scrambling to figure out how to remove. You can buy a shower filter for about $30 at most health food stores. You just screw it onto the shower's water source between the pipe coming out of the wall and the shower head itself and you're done. You can even buy replacement filters for less so you don't have to buy a new filter system every time.

These shower filters usually run the water through carbon. We already know how that won't remove enough chlorine and fluoride to make water suitable for drinking. In this regard, we know these shower filters are not likely removing all the chemicals from the water. But with such an easy and inexpensive step, you can at least begin to reduce the amount of chemicals in your showering experience. For a lot of people, this simple step can reduce the load on their bodies and bring some relief. I hope I didn't scare you away from showering and your plan is to simply stink from now on.

Microwaves

Much of this book has been about correcting issues to allow your body to use the food you're eating and to improve its ability to remove junk and synthetic substances that your body can't process. That's why microwaves are an important topic. If you're going to correct your digestion so that you can actually pull the nutrients out of the food you eat, the food you eat should be something that your body can use. Too many sources have scared me away from using microwaves. It is believed that the way microwaves heat food is a process that changes the molecular structure of the food in order to create the friction that makes it hot. When you change the molecular structure of a natural food, it can become unrecognizable to the body and the body may not be able to process it correctly.

There are as many studies that show this to be false as there are studies that show this problem to be true. Is it easier to heat something in the microwave? Of course it is. But you need to understand: If anything heated by a microwave not only loses its nutritional value to the body, but also becomes a problem that the body has to deal with, that is not worth the risk to me. It will take you longer to prepare your food without a microwave; but it could be time that you save in the long run by reducing the number of doctor and hospital visits you need to make. I just use my microwave as a very fancy clock.

You may still be skeptical and thinking, "Okay Tony, I'll fix my digestion, but why ya gotta mess with my Hot Pockets?" I'll give you a little experiment. Go down to Home Depot and buy two identical potted plants. Name one plant "Ricky" and the other one "Reject Bastard-Child." I guess you can pick your own names if you want. In any case, take them home and put them in the same light. Water one plant with normal water, and the other plant with water that has been microwaved. Don't pour the hot water in the plant because obviously that won't go well. Just microwave some water and let it cool to room temperature before you water with it.

At the end of your experiment, I think you will find that one plant is happy, while the other plant has earned the name I suggested. Many believe that microwaves can even change the structure of water and turn it into an evil substance.

Many chain restaurants have switched over to cooking all of their food in microwaves. Food is shipped in bags and the "cooks" simply pop the bags in the microwave. The only cooking they do is in the deep fryer. Are ya kiddin' me? If I was in the boardroom when they made that decision, you would have heard a world of cussing.

What Am I Cooking In?

To keep this brief, understand that what you cook with counts. If you're cooking in plastics, aluminum, or typical "non-stick" cookware, some of these poisons are off-gassing into your food and into your body. This creates another toxin that your body has to deal with. Some of these heavy metal toxins don't have an exit strategy from the body and can accumulate and cause all types of trouble. Glass is always safe to cook with or drink out of, stainless steel is rarely suspect (with the idea that magnetic stainless steel is best since it won't deliver significant amounts of nickel into the food). Enamel cookware is also considered to be safer than most non-stick cookware.

What's In My Mouth?

The medical field is not the only world that practically gives us a "daily allowance" of toxins. We learned in the middle of the 18th century that mercury is poison and nothing has changed since—mercury is still poison. After the dentist finishes putting mercury into someone's teeth, he takes what is left over and puts it in a special container marked "hazardous materials." That container then goes into another container marked "hazardous materials." Next, a little truck that has the special markings and permits required to haul hazardous materials comes and picks up that mercury from the dentist's office. And of course the ADA doctors will still tell you it's safe to put mercury in your mouth and let it seep into your head 24 hours a day. Dental work that is toxic, medications that are toxic—with all this disclosure I feel like I'm breaking the news to Honey Boo Boo that there is no Easter Bunny.

Smoking

Smoking? Seriously? I don't really need to explain this, do I? I think you understand that you'll need to stop smoking to have any chance of improving your health. People think that smoking just affects the lungs; but it also puts a lot of tar and chemicals in the body that need to be filtered out by the liver. As I said in an earlier chapter, the two most important factors in health, in my opinion, are digestion and liver function. We aren't what we eat—we are what we can assimilate and what we can't remove. If your liver is overwhelmed, the body is having a hard time removing all the junk that should be removed. If it can't be removed, the junk will be stored in joints, tissues, or fat cells.

Here's the good news: The people who have a difficult time trying to quit smoking are almost always people with a low mineral content. The nicotine and the chemicals thicken blood and constrict the vascular system to raise blood pressure. So, when people with no mineral identity try to quit, it can sometimes be hard for them because smoking was helping to lift their blood pressure. If you are a smoker and your *Imbalance Guide* shows that you may be dealing with an Electrolyte Deficiency Imbalance, losing the smokes might just be a whole lot easier when you improve this imbalance. You're still going to have to want to quit. It's not going to be magic, but it will make it physiologically easier. Understanding how the body works can change the viewpoint of choices that we make in our lives. This new understanding can reveal that a bad habit could actually be a form of self-medication. The exciting part is that the bad habit is easier to get rid of when it no longer represents the main choice for the "medication." To learn more, go to www.KickItNaturally.com and type "How to Quit Smoking" in the search box. You will find the link to our podcast episode on this topic.

Antibiotics

Antibiotics don't just break apart the bad bacteria in your body; they also break apart all the good bacteria that live in your intestines. These good bacteria do these good things: Help with digestion, control infestation from yeast and bad bacteria like candida, make the B vitamins we need, and help clean putrefied fecal matter off colon walls. When we take antibiotics and wipe out all the good bacteria along with the bad, we need to replace the good bacteria with probiotics. Yet our doctors don't normally teach us how to do this.

Here's another issue many people, like me, have with antibiotics: Many antibiotics are actually made from fungus. When you use these antibiotics to break apart a bacterial issue or improve a viral problem, you're actually setting up the terrain of the body in a way that allows fungal problems to flourish. Imagine you have a garden and weeds are taking over in a big way. Would you try to eliminate those weeds by planting new weeds that were designed to kill the original weeds? That sentence alone sounds horribly dumb just from the number of times "weeds" showed up. If the sentence sounds stupid, obviously the idea is not that brilliant. If you want to get rid of a problem, it might be a good idea to use a method that isn't going to end up creating another problem.

Flu Shots

Ignorant.

Alkalizing Water And Water Filters

In the marketplace today, there is a lot of information about "alkalizing" that is a heaping pile of fiction. I don't cover the Acid and Alkaline Imbalances in this book, but I do include them in Appendix C. However, if you are currently using, or plan to use any alkalizing products or alkalizing water, be sure to read about them in Appendix C. It's very important that you understand if these products are right for you or not.

More About Tony

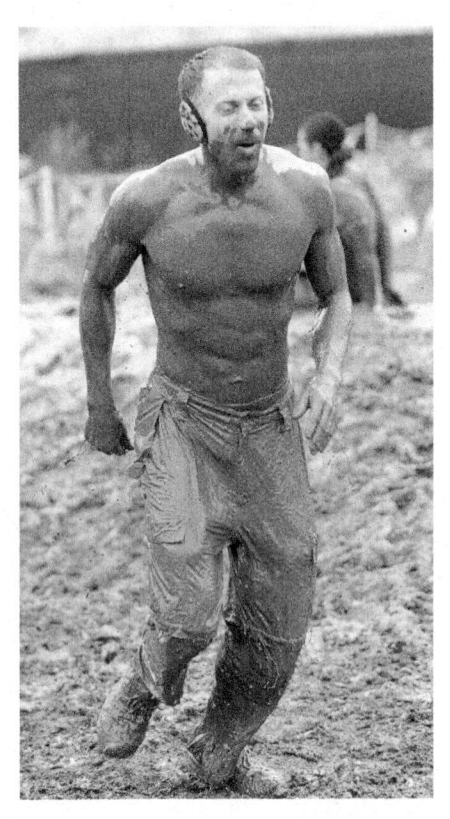

Like most natural health experts, Tony began his career in stand-up comedy. Touring professionally as a comic for nearly a decade, he never envisioned that he would one day teach the world how to sleep, poop, and even lose weight.

On Valentine's Day, 2004, Tony lost his voice and it didn't came back. After twenty-three doctors couldn't figure out the problem, Tony decided it was time to dig for his own answers. Eight years later, not only did Tony figure out his own issues, he also happened upon hidden information about how to improve countless other health problems.

Though Tony likes to boast about the fact that he holds no legitimate credentials (nor does he believe that we need any more "experts" from the same pool of knowledge already failing so many with health issues), he is greatly respected by his peers in the natural health industry. The biggest manufacturers in the health, fitness and organic products industries send Tony their products every year in hopes of winning one of his GearAwards.

Beyond working with many celebrity clients, Tony is on the executive board of *The Coalition for Health Education*, a nonprofit association that helps professionals and their clients learn about health through nutrition. Additionally, Tony teaches monthly webinars about nutrition to doctors, nutritionists and other health care professionals from more than thirty-five countries.

You can also find Tony producing documentaries like the upcoming, *Why Am I So Fat?* A film that teaches the truth about weight loss while showcasing Tony's client, Gabe Evans, who lost 200 pounds in 9 ½ months by treating Tony's word as gospel.

To learn more about Tony, visit www.KickItNaturally.com

REFERENCES

Chapter 1: Hi

Chimonas S, Evarts SD, Littlehale SK, Rothman DJ. Managing conflicts of interest in clinical care: the "race to the middle" at U.S. medical schools. *Acad Med*. 2013 Oct;88(10):1464-70. doi: 10.1097/ACM.0b013e3182a2e204.

Harrison C. US Patent Office issues guidelines on natural product patent eligibility. *Nat Rev Drug Discov*. 2014 Apr;13(4):250. doi: 10.1038/nrd4303.

Aceto JF. Patent portfolios after myriad, how to fit in those new genes. *ACS Med Chem Lett*. 2013 Jul 12;4(8):681-3.

Sloss A, Kubler P. Prescribing in liver disease. *Aust Presc*. 2009;32:32-5

Wilkinson GR, Shand DG. Commentary: a physiological approach to hepatic drug clearance. *Clin Pharmacol Ther*. 1975 Oct;18(4):377-90.

Mitchell SJ, Hilmer SN. Drug-induced liver injury in older adults. *World J Gastroenterol*. 2007 Jan 21;13(3):329-40.

Andrade RJ, Robles M, Fernández-Castañer A, López-Ortega S, López-Vega MC, Lucena MI. Assessment of drug-induced hepatotoxicity in clinical practice: a challenge for gastroenterologists. *World J Gastroenterol*. 2007 Jan 21;13(3):329-40

Chapter 2: Seriously? I Just Wanna Poop & Chapter 3: Digestion

Untersmayr E, Jensen-Jarolim E. The role of protein digestibility and antacids on food allergy outcomes. *J Allergy Clin Immunol*. 2008 Jun;121(6):1301-8

Barrett J. POPs vs. Fat: Persistent Organic Pollutant Toxicity Targets and Is Modulated by Adipose Tissue, *Environ Health Perspect*. Feb 2013; 121(2): a61.

Evans D, Pye G, Bramley R, Clark AG, Dyson TJ, Hardcastle JD. Measurement of gastrointestinal pH profiles in normal ambulant human subjects. *Gut*. Aug 1988; 29(8): 1035–1041.

Fallingborg J. Intraluminal pH of the human gastrointestinal tract. *Dan Med Bull*. 1999 Jun;46(3):183-96.

Fallingborg J, Christensen LA, Ingeman-Nielsen M, Jacobsen BA, Abildgaard K, Rasmussen HH, Rasmussen SN. Measurement of gastrointestinal pH and regional transit times in normal children. *J Pediatr Gastroenterol Nutr.* 1990 Aug;11(2):211-4.

Kelly G. Hydrochloric Acid: Physiological Functions and Clinical Implications Alternative Medicine Review. Volume 2, Number 2. 1997, p.117

First Principles of Gastroenterology: The Basis of Disease and an Approach to Management, J.J Freeman & A.B.R. Tomson, p.177

Reshetnyak VI. Physiological and molecular biochemical mechanisms of bile formation. *World J Gastroenterol.* 2013 Nov 14;19(42):7341-60. doi: 10.3748/wjg.v19.i42.7341.

Sjöblom M, Singh AK, Zheng W, Wang J, Tuo B, Krabbenhöft A, Riederer B, Gros G, Seidler U. Duodenal acidity "sensing" but not epithelial HCO_3^- supply is critically dependent on carbonic anhydrase II expression. *Proc Natl Acad Sci U S A.* Aug 4, 2009; 106(31): 13094–13099

Allen A, Flemström G. Gastroduodenal mucus bicarbonate barrier: protection against acid and pepsin. *Amer Jour Phys* January 2005 Vol. 288

First Principles of Gastroenterology: The Basis of Disease and an Approach to Management, Fifth Edition, H.J. Freeman and A.B.R. Thomson, JANSSEN-ORTHO, p.193,197-209

Camilleri M, Parkman H, Shafi M, Abell T, Gerson L. Clinical Guideline: Management of Gastroparesis. *Am J Gastroenterol.* Jan 2013; 108(1): 18–38.

First Principles of Gastroenterology, 5th Edition: The Stomach and duodenum; B.J. Salena and R.H. Hunt, p.144

Cater RE 2nd (1992 Dec) The clinical importance of hypochlorhydria (a consequence of chronic Helicobacter infection): its possible etiological role in mineral and amino acid malabsorption, depression, and other syndromes *Med Hypotheses*; 39(4):375-83 PMID: 1494327.

McCarthy D. Adverse effects of proton pump inhibitor drugs: clues and conclusions. *Current Opinion in Gastroenterology.* November 2010, Volume 26, Issue 6; p 624–631

Prousky J. Is Vitamin B3 Dependency a Causal Factor in the Development of Hypochlorhydria and Achlorhydria? *The Journal of Orthomolecular Medicine* Vol. 16, 4th Quarter 2001

Hwang C, Ross V, Mahadevan U. Micronutrient deficiencies in inflammatory bowel disease: from A to zinc. *Inflamm Bowel Dis.* 2012 Oct;18(10):1961-81.

Recker RR. Calcium absorption and achlorhydria. *N Engl J Med*. 1985 Jul 11;313(2):70-3.

Heizer W. Normal and abnormal intestinal absorption by humans. *Environ Health Perspect*. Dec 1979; 33: 101–106.

Iwai W, Abe Y, Iijima K, Koike T, Uno K, Asano N, Imatani A, Shimosegawa T. Gastric hypochlorhydria is associated with an exacerbation of dyspeptic symptoms in female patients. *J Gastroenterol*. 2013 Feb;48(2):214-21.

Ostrow J, Resnick R. Hyperchlorhydria, duodenitis and duodenal ulcer: A clinical study of their interrelationships. *Ann Intern Med*. 1959;51(6):1303-1328. Hunt RH. The protective role of gastric acid. *Scand J Gastroenterol Suppl*. 1988;146:34-9.

Marshall BJ, Barrett LJ, Prakash C, McCallum R, Guerrant R, Urea Protects Helicobacter (Campylobacter) pylori From the Bactericial Effect of Acid. *Gasteroenterology*. 1990;99:697-762

Border J R. Multiple systems organ failure. *Ann Surg*. Aug 1992; 216(2): 111–116., p.114

Parsonnet J, Friedman GD. Helicobacter pylori infection and the risk of gastric carcinoma. *New England Journal of Medicine*, Oct. 17, 1991 - Vol 325, No.16; p.1127

Champagne ET. Low gastric hydrochloric acid secretion and mineral bioavailability. *Adv Exp Med Biol*. 1989;249:173-84.

Mackay JD, Bladon PT. Hypomagnesaemia due to proton-pump inhibitor therapy: a clinical case series. *Oxford Journals, QJM: An International Journal of Medicine*, Volume 103, Issue 6, Pp. 387-395

Champagne E. Low Gastric Hydrochloric Acid Secretion and Mineral Bioavailability: Mineral Absorption in the Monogastric GI Tract. *Advances in Experimental Medicine and Biology* Volume 249, 1989, pp 173-184

Davies RE, Roughton FJW. Hydrochloric acid production by isolated gastric mucosa *Biochem J*. 1948; 42(4): 609–621.

Zollner G, Trauner M. Mechanisms of cholestasis. *Clin Liver Dis*. 2008 Feb;12(1):1-26, vii.

Pratt DS. Cholestasis and cholestatic syndromes. *Curr Opin Gastroenterol*. 2005 May;21(3):270-4.

Alrefai WA, Gill RK. Bile acid transporters: structure, function, regulation and pathophysiological implications. *Pharm Res.* 2007 Oct;24(10):1803-23.

Scott-Conner CE, Grogan JB. The pathophysiology of biliary obstruction and its effect on phagocytic and immune function. *J Surg Res.* 1994 Aug;57(2):316-36.

Di Stefano M, Vos R, Vanuytsel T, Janssens J, Tack J. Prolonged duodenal acid perfusion and dyspeptic symptom occurrence in healthy volunteers. *Neurogastroenterology & Motility.* (2009) 21: 712–e40.

Freeman HJ, Thomson ABR. First Principles of Gastroenterology: The Basis of Disease and an Approach to Management, Fifth Edition. *Janssen-ortho,* p.192-209

Mowat A P, Arias, I M. . Liver function and oral contraceptives. (1969) *Journal of Reproduction Medicine,* 3, 19-29.

Boston Collaborative Drug Surveillance Programme (1973). Oral contraceptives and venous thromboembolic disease, surgically confirmed gallbladder disease and breast tumours. *Lancet,* 1,1399-1404.

Forker EL. The effect of estrogen on bile formation in the rat. *J Clin Invest.* 1969 Apr;48(4):654-63.

Somero G. Temperature adaptation of enzymes: biological optimization through structure-function compromises. *Annual Review of Ecology and Systematics* (1978): 1-29.

Thomson A, Keelan M. The aging gut. *Canadian Journal of Physiology and Pharmacology.* 1986, 64(1): 30-38.

Prasad AS. Clinical, endocrinologic, and biochemical effects of zinc deficiency. *Spec Top Endocrinol Metab.* 1985;7:45-76.

Chapter 4: Elimination & Digestion Gone Wild

Tontisirin K, Valyasevi A. Protein Energy Malnutrition Related to Diarrhea in Thai Children. *Journal of Nutritional Science and Vitaminology* Vol. 27 (1981) No. 6 P 513-520

PEM, PROTEIN ENERGY MALNUTRITION. "Protein Energy Malnutrition." Pediatric Clinics of North America, 2009

Dragstedt L, Dragstedt C, McClintock J, Chase C S. A study of the factors involved in the production and absorption of toxic materials from the intestine. *J Exp Med.* Aug 1, 1919; 30(2): 109–121.

Pathological Physiology of Internal Diseases, By Albion Walter Hewlett, New York And London D. Appleton & Company, 1917, p.146

Nutrition and Diagnosis-related Care, 6th Edition, By Sylvia Escott-Stump, p.471

Layer P, Keller J. Pancreatic enzymes: secretion and luminal nutrient digestion in health and disease. *J Clin Gastroenterol*. 1999 Jan;28(1):3-10.

Rosado JL, Solomons NW, Lisker R, Bourges H. Enzyme replacement therapy for primary adult lactase deficiency. Effective reduction of lactose malabsorption and milk intolerance by direct addition of beta-galactosidase to milk at mealtime. *Gastroenterology*. 1984 Nov;87(5):1072-82.

Faria AM, Gomes-Santos AC, Gonçalves JL, Moreira TG, Medeiros SR, Dourado LP, Cara DC. Food components and the immune system: from tonic agents to allergens. *Front Immunol*. 2013 May 17;4:102.

Chapter 5: Simple Self-Testing & Chapter 6: Understanding Your Biological Individuality

Guyton A. Blood Pressure Control-Special Role of the Kidneys and Body Fluids. *Science* 252.5014 (Jun 28, 1991): 1813.

Knochel JP. Neuromuscular manifestations of electrolyte disorders. *Am J Med*. 1982 Mar;72(3):521-35.

Riggs JE. Neurologic manifestations of electrolyte disturbances. *Neurol Clin*. 2002 Feb;20(1):227-39, vii.

Weiner M, Epstein FH. Signs and symptoms of electrolyte disorders. *Yale J Biol Med*. 1970 Oct;43(2):76-109.

Mäestu J, Eliakim A, Jürimäe J, Valter I, Jürimäe T. Anabolic and catabolic hormones and energy balance of the male bodybuilders during the preparation for the competition. *J Strength Cond Res*. 2010 Apr;24(4):1074-81.

The Doctor Who Cures Cancer. William Kelley. Be Well Books, 1996

An Analytical System of Clinical Nutrition. Guy Schenker. P. 235

Brooks G, Mercier J. Balance of carbohydrate and lipid utilization during exercise: the "crossover" concept. *Journal of Applied Physiology* June 1994 Vol. 76 no. 6, 2253-2261

Scheutz F, Poulsen S. Determining causation in epidemiology. *Community Dent Oral Epidemiol*. 1999 Jun;27(3):161-70.

Bättig B, Steiner A, Jeck T, Vetter W. Blood pressure self-measurement in normotensive and hypertensive patients. Journal of Hypertension. *Supplement: Official Journal of the International Society of Hypertension* [1989, 7(3):S59-63]

Louie AK, Louie EK, Lannon RA. Systemic hypertension associated with tricyclic antidepressant treatment in patients with panic disorder. *Am J Cardiol*. 1992 Nov

15;70(15):1306-9.

Grodins FS. Respiration and the regulation of acid-base balance. *AMA Arch Intern Med*. 1957 Apr;99(4):569-72.

Chapter 7: How Imbalances Contribute To Constipation

Mitchell P. Foundations of vectorial metabolism and osmochemistry. *Biosci Rep*. 1991 Dec;11(6):297-344; discussion 345-6.

Oliver W J. Sodium Homeostasis and Low Blood Pressure Populations Epidemiology of Arterial Blood Pressure. *Developments in Cardiovascular Medicine*. Volume 8, 1980, pp 229-241

Gomez T, Molé P, Collins A. Dilution of body fluid electrolytes affects bioelectrical impedance measurements. *Research in Sports Medicine An International Journal* 4(4):291-298 · December 1993

Cravioto J, Delicardie ER. Mental performance in school age children. Findings after recovery from early severe malnutrition. *Am J Dis Child*. 1970 Nov;120(5):404-10.

Sandstead H. Nutrition and Brain Function: Trace Elements. *Nutrition Reviews* Volume 44, Issue Supplement s3, pages 37–41, May 1986

Watson G, Comrey A. Nutritional replacement for mental illness. *Psychol.*, 1954, 38, 25 1-264.

Kellum J A. Determinants of blood pH in health and disease . *Critical Care* 2000, 4:6-14

Electrolytes Disturbances and Seizures. Luis Castilla-Guerra, María del Carmen Fernández-Moreno, José Manuel López-Chozas and Ricardo Fernández-Bolaños

Rhoades J D. Salinity: Electrical Conductivity and Total Dissolved Solids. Methods of Soil Analysis Part 3—Chemical Methods

Brown RT, Polinsky RJ, Lee GK, Deeter JA. Insulin-induced hypotension and neurogenic orthostatic hypotension. *Neurology*. 1986 Oct;36(10):1402-6.

Kobori H, Nangaku M, Navar LG, Nishiyama A. The intrarenal renin-angiotensin system: from physiology to the pathobiology of hypertension and kidney disease. *Pharmacol Rev*. 2007 Sep;59(3):251-87.

Engelmann W, Schrempf M. Membrane Models for Circadian Rhythms. *Photochemical and Photobiological Reviews* 1980, pp 49-86

Revici E. Research in Pathophysiology as Basis for Guided Chemotherapy, with Special Application to Cancer. Princeton, NJ: D. Van Nostrand Company, 1961.

Alenghat FJ, Golan DE. Membrane protein dynamics and functional implications in mammalian cells. *Curr Top Membr*. 2013;72:89-120.

Brinkmann K. Circadian rhythm in the kinetics of acid denaturation of cell membranes of Euglena gracilis. *Planta* (Berlin)1976a, 129:221–227.

Carrasco L. The inhibition of cell functions after viral infection. 1977, *FEBS Lett.* 76:11–15

Eskin A, Corrent G. Effects of divalent cations and metabolic poisons on the circadian rhythm from the Aplysia eye. *J. Comp. Physiol.* 1977, **117**:1–21.

Cummings F W. A biochemical model of the circadian clock. 1975, *J. Theor. Biol.* 55:455–470.

Aldridge J. Short-range intercellular communication, biochemical oscillations and circadian rhythms. *Handbook of Engineering in Medicine and Biology* (1976): 55-147.

Adam K. Sleep as a restorative process and a theory to explain why. *Prog Brain Res*. 1980;53:289-305.

Papahadjopoulos D. Cholesterol and cell membrane function: A hypothesis concerning the etiology of atherosclerosis. *Journal of Theoretical Biology* Volume 43, Issue 2, February 1974, Pages 329–337

Erecińska M, Wilson D F. Regulation of cellular energy metabolism. *The Journal of Membrane Biology* 1982, Volume 70, Issue 1, pp 1-14

Ginsberg L, Gershfeld N L. Membrane bilayer instability and the pathogenesis of disorders of myelin. *Neurosci Lett.* 1991 Sep 2;130(1):133-6.

Caroli A, Del Favero G, Di Mario F. Lipid pattern and plasma insulin in diabetics with gall stones. *Gut* 32.3 (1991): 339-340.

Ravussin E, Smith SR, Ann N Y. Increased fat intake, impaired fat oxidation, and failure of fat cell proliferation result in ectopic fat storage, insulin resistance, and type 2 diabetes mellitus. *Acad Sci*. 2002 Jun;967:363-78.

Teff KL, Grudziak J, Townsend RR, Dunn TN, Grant RW, Adams SH, Keim NL, Cummings BP, Stanhope KL, Havel PJ. Endocrine and metabolic effects of consuming fructose- and glucose-sweetened beverages with meals in obese men and women: influence of insulin resistance on plasma triglyceride responses. *J Clin Endocrinol Metab*. 2009 May;94(5):1562-9.

Chapter 8: What Else Can Help?

Stormont J, Waterhouse C. The Genesis of Hyponatremia Associated with Marked Overhydration and Water Intoxication. *Circulation*. 1961; 24: 191-203

Yamashiro M, Hasegawa H, Matsuda A, Kinoshita M, Matsumura O, Isoda K, Mitarai T. A case of water intoxication with prolonged hyponatremia caused by excessive water drinking and secondary SIADH. *Case Rep Nephrol Urol*. 2013 Dec 21;3(2):147-52.

Callaham M. Panic disorders, hyperventilation, and the dreaded brown paper bag. *Ann Emerg Med*. 1997 Dec;30(6):838.

Consumption of soft drinks with phosphoric acid as a risk factor for the development of hypocalcemia in children: A case-control study, *The Journal of Pediatrics* Volume 126, Issue 6, June 1995, Pages 940–942.

Lindseth GN, Coolahan SE, Petros TV, Lindseth PD. Neurobehavioral effects of aspartame consumption. *Res Nurs Health*. 2014 Jun;37(3):185-93.

Humphries P, Pretorius E, Naudé H. Direct and indirect cellular effects of aspartame on the brain. *Eur J Clin Nutr*. 2008 Apr;62(4):451-62.

Coulombe RA Jr, Sharma RP. Neurobiochemical alterations induced by the artificial sweetener aspartame (NutraSweet). *Toxicol Appl Pharmacol*. 1986 Mar 30;83(1):79-85.

Cheremisinoff, Nicholas P. *Practical guide to industrial safety: methods for process safety professionals*. CRC Press, 2000.

Schneeman BO. Fiber, inulin and oligofructose: similarities and differences. *J Nutr*. 1999 Jul;129(7 Suppl):1424S-7S.

Jong-Sik J,Jong-Hyun L. Phytochemical and pharmacological aspects of *Siraitia grosvenorii*, luo han kuo. *Oriental Pharmacy and Experimental Medicine* December 2012, Volume 12, Issue 4, pp 233-239

McCowen K, Malhotra A, Bistrian B R. Stress-Induced Hyperglycemia. *Critical Care Clinics* Volume 17, Issue 1, 1 January 2001, Pages 107–124

Kopelman TR, O'Neill PJ, Kanneganti SR, Davis KM, Drachman DA. The relationship of plasma glucose and glycosylated hemoglobin A1C levels among nondiabetic trauma patients. *Trauma*. 2008 Jan;64(1):30-3; discussion 33-4.

Taché Y, Perdue MH. Role of peripheral CRF signalling pathways in stress-related alterations of gut motility and mucosal function. *Neurogastroenterol Motil*. 2004 Apr;16 Suppl 1:137-42.

Taché Y, Martinez V, Million M, Maillot C. Role of corticotropin releasing factor receptor subtype 1 in stress-related functional colonic alterations: implications in irritable bowel syndrome. *Eur J Surg Suppl*. 2002;(587):16-22.

Frayn K N. Hormonal Control of Metabolism in Trauma and Sepsis. *Clinical Endocrinology*, Volume 24, Issue 5, pages 577–599, May 1986

Chapter 9: Foods Specific To You & Chapter 10: Supplements That Could Help

Diesendorf M, Colquhoun J, Spittle BJ, Everingham DN, Clutterbuck FW. New evidence on fluoridation. *Aust N Z J Public Health*. 1997 Apr;21(2):187-90.

McDonald TA, Komulainen H. Carcinogenicity of the chlorination disinfection by-product MX. *J Environ Sci Health C Environ Carcinog Ecotoxicol Rev*. 2005;23(2):163-214.

Coplan MJ, Patch SC, Masters RD, Bachman MS. Confirmation of and explanations for elevated blood lead and other disorders in children exposed to water disinfection and fluoridation chemicals. *Neurotoxicology*. 2007 Sep;28(5):1032-42. Epub 2007 Mar 1

Newsholme P, Procopio J, Lima M, Pithon-Curi T C, Curi R. Glutamine and glutamate-their central role on cell metabolism and function. *Cell Bio & Func*. 2002

Chapter 11: Case Studies & FAQs

Fallingborg J. Intraluminal pH of the human gastrointestinal tract. *Dan Med Bull*. 1999 Jun;46(3):183-96.

Fallingborg J, Christensen LA, Ingeman-Nielsen M, Jacobsen BA, Abildgaard K, Rasmussen HH, Rasmussen SN. Measurement of gastrointestinal pH and regional transit times in normal children. *J Pediatr Gastroenterol Nutr*. 1990 Aug;11(2):211-4.

Kelly G. Hydrochloric Acid: Physiological Functions and Clinical Implications Alternative Medicine Review. Volume 2, Number 2. 1997, p.117

Davies RE, Roughton FJW. Hydrochloric acid production by isolated gastric mucosa *Biochem J*. 1948; 42(4): 609–621.

Zollner G, Trauner M. Mechanisms of cholestasis. *Clin Liver Dis*. 2008 Feb;12(1):1-26, vii.

Pratt DS. Cholestasis and cholestatic syndromes. *Curr Opin Gastroenterol*. 2005 May;21(3):270-4.

Alrefai WA, Gill RK. Bile acid transporters: structure, function, regulation and pathophysiological implications. *Pharm Res*. 2007 Oct;24(10):1803-23.

Chapter 12 (The Sum Up): Review & Make Your Plan

Kelly G. Hydrochloric Acid: Physiological Functions and Clinical Implications Alternative Medicine Review. Volume 2, Number 2. 1997, p.117

Davies RE, Roughton FJW. Hydrochloric acid production by isolated gastric mucosa *Biochem J*. 1948; 42(4): 609–621.

Pratt DS. Cholestasis and cholestatic syndromes. *Curr Opin Gastroenterol*. 2005 May;21(3):270-4.

That's it. Close the book now.

Printed in Great Britain
by Amazon